SEXUAL HEALTH AWARENESS

What Are Urinary Tract Infections?

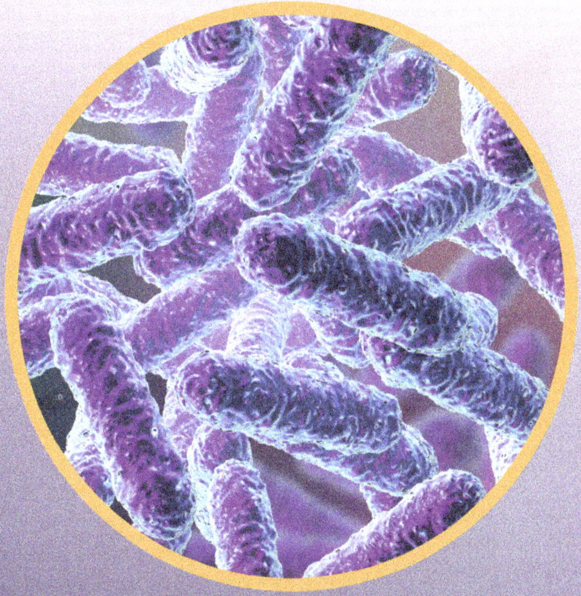

Sadie Silva

ROSEN PUBLISHING
NEW YORK

Published in 2022 by The Rosen Publishing Group, Inc.
29 East 21st Street, New York, NY 10010

First Edition

Portions of this work were originally authored by Susan Henneberg and published as *Your Sexual Health: UTI.* All new material in this edition was authored by Sadie Silva.

Library of Congress Cataloging-in-Publication Data

Names: Silva, Sadie, author.
Title: What are urinary tract infections? / Sadie Silva.
Description: New York : Rosen Publishing Group, [2022] | Series: Sexual health awareness | Includes index.
Identifiers: LCCN 2021029139 (print) | LCCN 2021029140 (ebook) | ISBN 9781499472165 (library binding) | ISBN 9781499472158 (paperback) | ISBN 9781499472172 (ebook)
Subjects: LCSH: Urinary tract infections.
Classification: LCC RC901.8 .S55 2022 (print) | LCC RC901.8 (ebook) | DDC 616.6--dc23
LC record available at https://lccn.loc.gov/2021029139
LC ebook record available at https://lccn.loc.gov/2021029140

Manufactured in the United States of America

CPSIA Compliance Information: Batch #CWRYA22. For further information contact Rosen Publishing, New York, New York at 1-800-237-9932.

CONTENTS

INTRODUCTION

There's never a good time for a urinary tract infection (UTI) to show up. These infections are very common, and in some cases, very serious. You may notice a strong urge to pee that doesn't go away, no matter how many trips you take to the bathroom. When you do pee, it might burn. Your urine might be cloudy, discolored, or strong smelling. And you might have pain in your pelvis. If you or someone you know has these symptoms, it's important to take action to diagnose and treat your UTI.

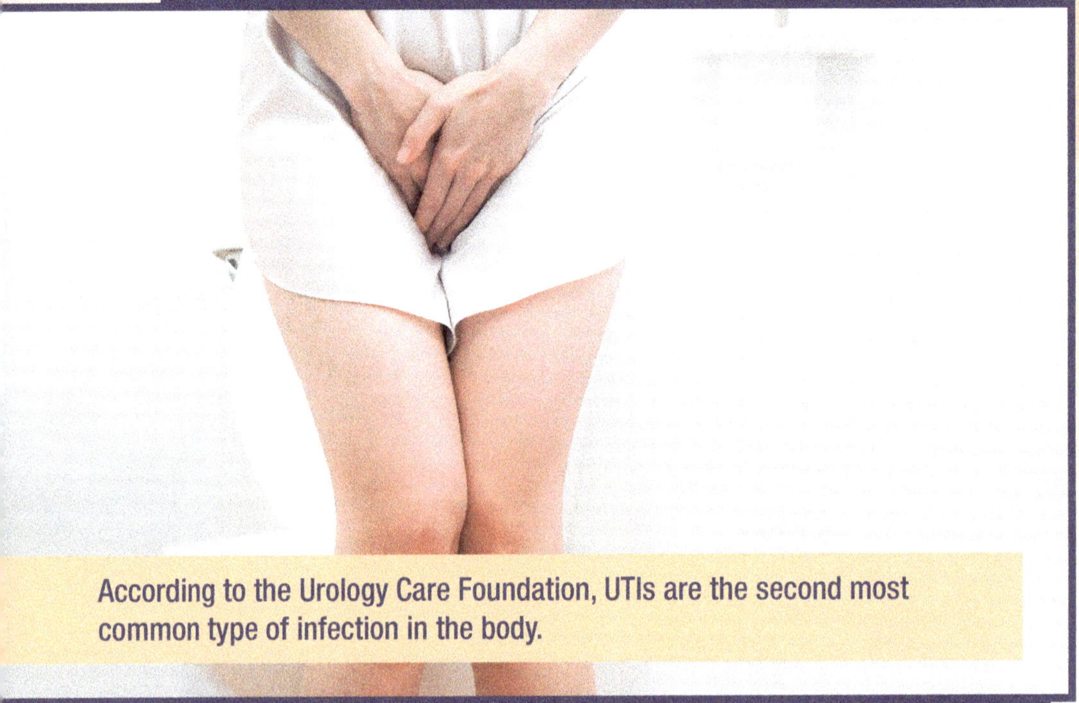

According to the Urology Care Foundation, UTIs are the second most common type of infection in the body.

More than 8 million doctor visits each year occur because of UTIs. These infections impact about 10 in 25 biologically female individuals and 3 in 25 biologically male individuals in their lifetime. Some people get recurrent UTIs, which means three or more each year. A urinary tract infection is one of the most common reasons why teens, especially biologically female teens, visit the doctor. And while UTIs in biological males are rarer, they are often more serious than those in biological females. Since the structure of the male and female urinary tract is different, your assigned sex (a label based on your hormones, chromosomes, and genitals at birth) plays a large role in the likelihood of your developing a UTI, regardless of gender identity.

UTIs also have to do with your sexual health. Biologically female individuals may have increased UTIs starting in puberty and later after they reach menopause. This is sometimes because of hormonal changes during these periods of life. Some link the onset of UTIs in puberty with the onset of sexual activity. What's the connection? Having sex is one of the most common ways that harmful bacteria find their way into a female's urethra. But it's not the only way. Because of female anatomy, UTIs can happen to biologically female individuals for a variety of reasons.

It's important to have UTIs treated by a doctor. They are quickly diagnosed with a urine sample and are usually easily treated with antibiotics. Modern technology has increased doctors' ability to prescribe the right antibiotic for the particular strain of bacteria a patient may have. Until the infection clears up, a person with a UTI needs to rest, drink lots of fluids, and take over-the-counter pain medications. If a UTI isn't treated, it can become a kidney infection, which is a more serious condition.

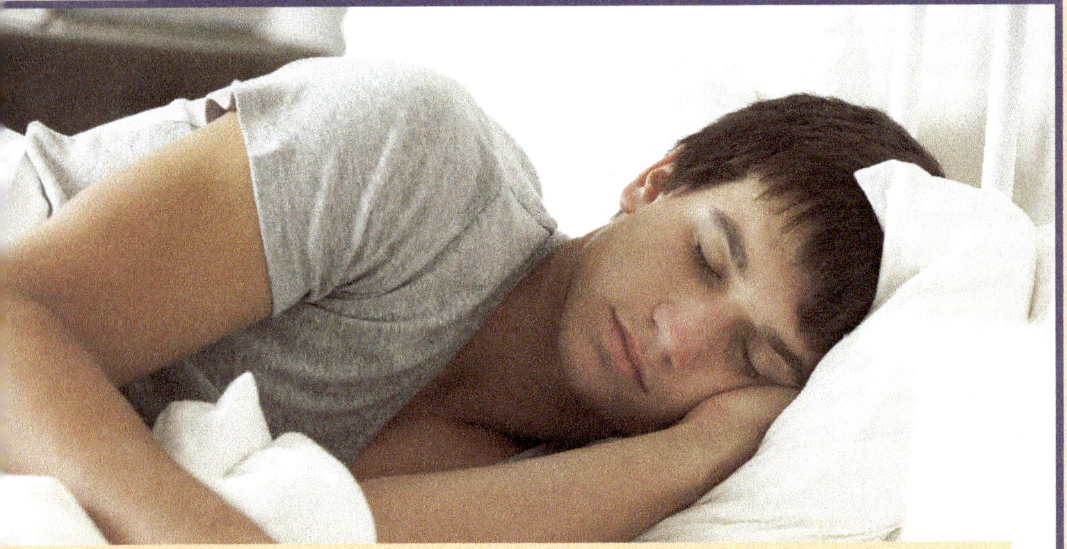

Rest is a major part of treating a UTI. It's important to get the recommended amount of sleep and not put your body through too much stress.

Some people are embarrassed to have a UTI, since it means you'll have to use the bathroom a lot. Teens might even feel ashamed of a UTI because of stigmas around sexual activity. While those feelings are valid, it's important to know that your health is the number-one priority. That might mean advocating for your health to doctors, school nurses, parents, teachers, and coaches. Learning about UTIs and making the best choices for your physical and mental health are necessary steps toward reclaiming your well-being.

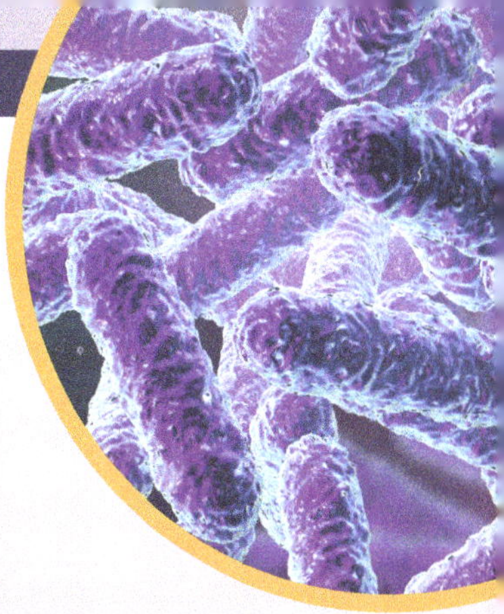

CHAPTER 1

HELLO, URINARY TRACT INFECTION

The first time you get a UTI, you might have no idea what's going on. Usually, people can pee without a problem, and we take that for granted. You may not even know what your urinary tract is until it's not working properly.

The urinary tract plays an important role in the body. It's your body's drainage system for urine. Urine is a way for your body to regulate the amount of water in your body. Excess water is eliminated as urine. But urine is more than just the water you drink. It's also made up of salt, a chemical called ammonia, and waste products such as urea and creatinine. The urine travels through the urinary tract on its way out of your body. The urinary tract is a pathway that includes several important organs.

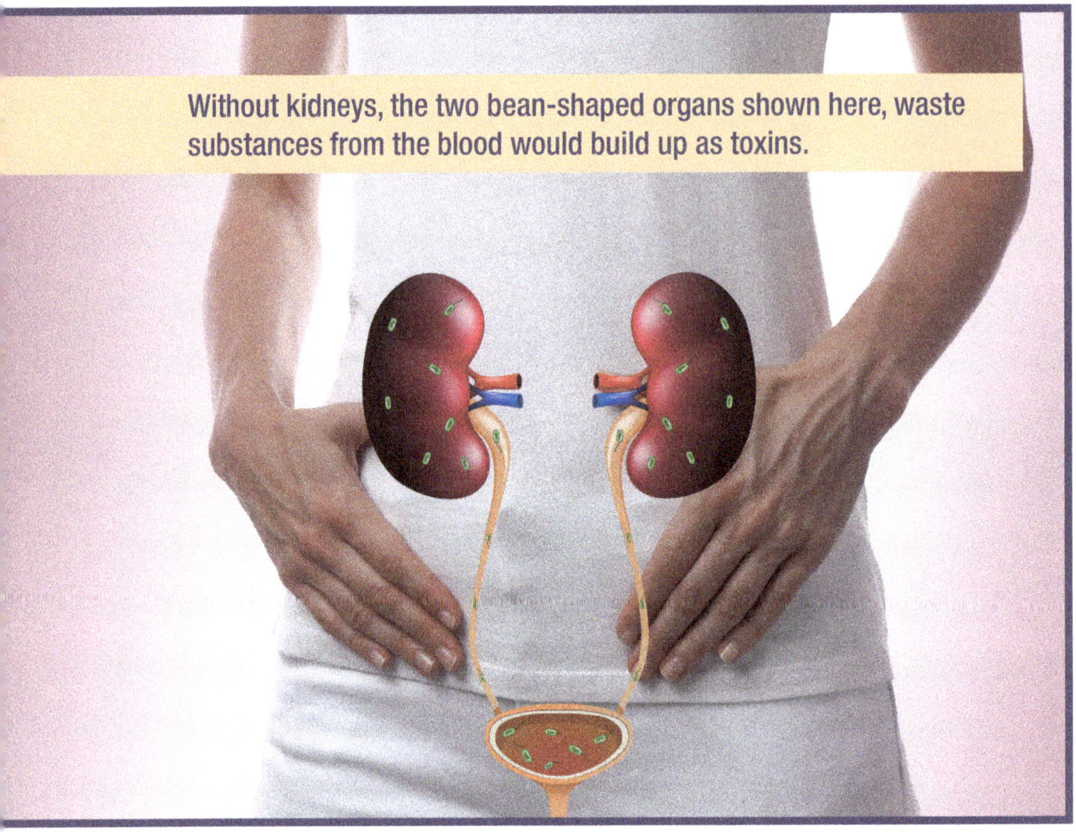

Without kidneys, the two bean-shaped organs shown here, waste substances from the blood would build up as toxins.

Your two kidneys filter waste substances from the blood and produce urine to get rid of them. The ureters are thin tubes that take urine from the kidneys to the bladder. The bladder holds the urine until it's time to go to the bathroom. The urethra is the tube that carries urine from the bladder out of the body.

Different types of UTIs occur in different parts of the urinary tract. Upper urinary tract infections involve the kidneys and ureters, while lower urinary tract infections involve the bladder and urethra. Biological females have more lower urinary tract infections than males. As you'll find out, the structure and functioning of your urinary tract has a lot to do with your urinary health.

DIFFERENT SEXES, DIFFERENT SYSTEMS

Male and female urinary systems have the same basic organs and purpose. However, differences between the systems can lead to differences in the prevalence and severity of UTIs.

People who are biologically female have short urethras. The urethra's only purpose is to take urine from the bladder out of the body. The opening of the urethra is close to the anus, the outlet for the digestive system. The urethra is also close to the vagina. The position of the opening of the urethra close to the anus and vagina makes it easier for bacteria to travel these short distances. That's why those with this structure get more infections in their urinary tracts than others.

People who are biologically male share their urinary system with their reproductive system. Their urethras are longer than those of others. The male urethra extends through the penis. It's also responsible for ejaculating, or ejecting, semen through the penis. Because of the long male urethra and its distance from the anus, it's harder for bacteria to get into the urinary tract. That's why those are biologically male have fewer UTIs.

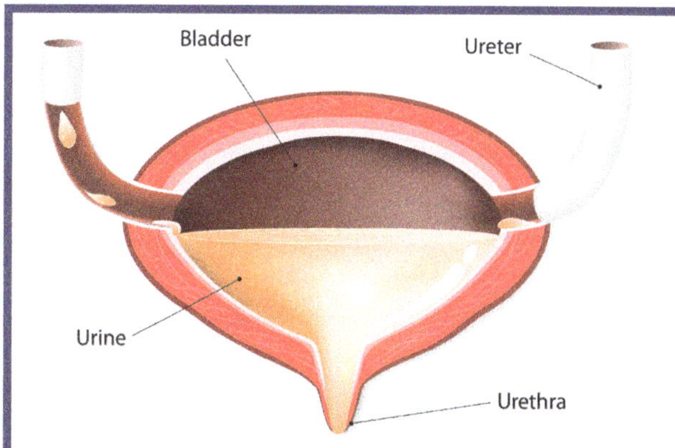

This diagram shows urine inside of the bladder and how it empties through the urethra.

FINDING THE CULPRIT

If you feel an intense need to pee constantly, burning when you pee, or pelvic pain, you'll probably want to figure out the cause. After you describe your symptoms to a doctor, they'll likely know the culprit—a UTI. That's because it's so common. However, the doctor will still test your urine to make sure their guess is correct.

The doctor will probably ask you for a urine sample. In addition to the normal waste products usually filtered by the kidneys, your urine will also contain bacteria. Bacteria are microbes so small they can be seen only with a microscope. This bacteria, usually *E. coli*, may have traveled up through the urethra and infected the bladder, causing a bladder infection, or cystitis.

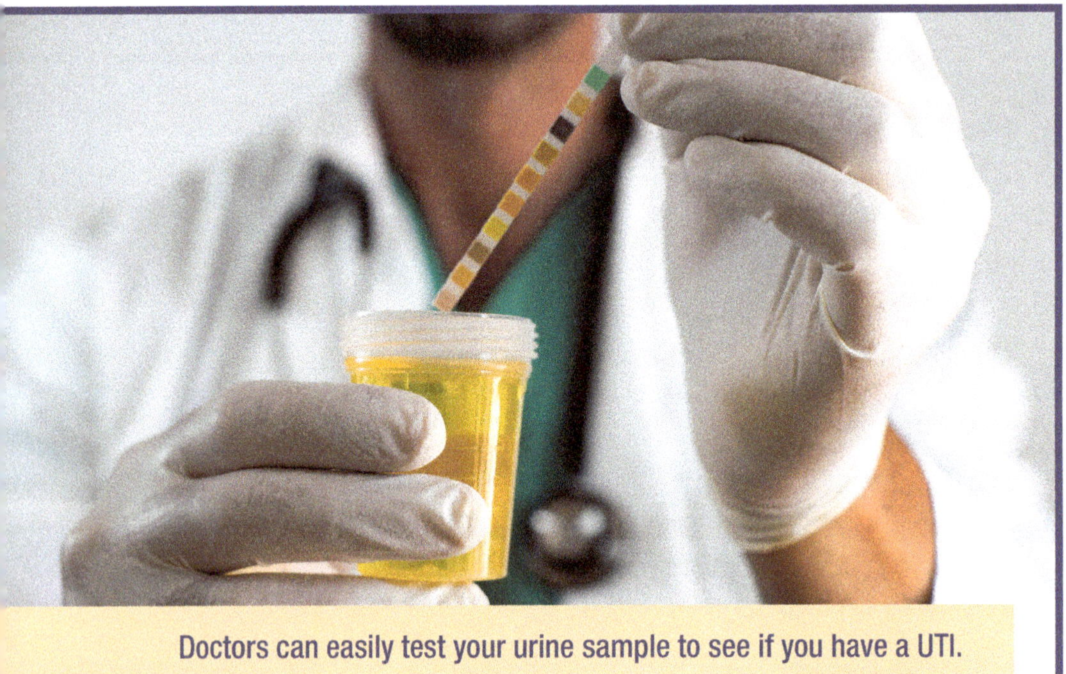

Doctors can easily test your urine sample to see if you have a UTI.

The bladder wall is irritated by the bacteria, causing pain. Bacteria can also infect the urethra, resulting in urethritis. It can infect the kidneys, which causes pyelonephritis, a more serious disease. If you have back pain, high fever, and vomiting, you might have a kidney infection.

BAD BACTERIA

What's *E. coli*, anyway? You've probably heard of *E. coli* because some forms of it cause infections. *E. coli* is the shortened name of a bacteria called *Escherichia coli*. *E. coli* lives in your intestines. While most types of this bacteria are harmless, others are bad bacteria that can make you sick. One way you can get *E. coli* infections is by eating food that's gone bad or has been contaminated. People who are traveling to a new place may get "traveler's diarrhea," which is picked up by eating or drinking contaminated foods. You can also get it from contaminated drinking water, contact with a person who has it, contaminated swimming water, and petting zoos. If you are exposed to this kind of *E. coli*, you may start to be sick between one day and one week later. You might have diarrhea, cramping and pain in the stomach, nausea, and vomiting. Every body reacts to it differently, but some severe cases can cause kidney failure or death.

You can avoid getting sick from *E. coli* by washing your hands frequently with soap. You can also wash produce, cook food according to CDC guidelines for temperature, and keep a clean cooking area. You can prevent a UTI from *E. coli* by following basic sexual health practices and other hygiene practices.

SEX AND UTIS

UTIs have many causes. People with biologically female anatomy may get it from wiping back to front after a bowel movement, sending bacteria to the urethra. People may get it from not peeing frequently enough when they have to. However, because it's a common cause, sex and UTIs are often linked in people's minds. Because of this, there has been a stigma around UTIs, with some people even calling it the "honeymoon disease." Understanding how sex and UTIs are linked can help you take control of your health.

Having sex can push bacteria from the vaginal area into the urethral opening. Switching between anal and vaginal sex without cleaning in between can cause bits of feces to get near the urethra. This is why people who are sexually active can get UTIs more often. These types of infections aren't contagious, so you can't catch a UTI from someone else. Still, you'll want to be honest with your sexual partner if you have a UTI, since sex isn't recommended while you're recovering from one.

Sometimes different methods of contraception can cause a UTI. That's one reason why finding the best form of contraception for your body is important. Using a spermicide, such as contraceptive creams, jellies, sponges, and foams, during sex can increase your chances of getting a UTI. The purpose of spermicides is to kill sperm during sex to prevent pregnancy. Spermicides can also kill off naturally occurring good bacteria that protect against invading bad bacteria. The invading bacteria are able to establish colonies and create infection.

Women who use diaphragms are at an increased risk for UTIs. They usually use them with spermicidal jelly or cream. Another reason diaphragms may cause UTIs is that they push up against the urethra, making it harder to fully empty the bladder. The urine that is left can grow bacteria.

One useful tip for avoiding UTIs while you're sexually active is to pee before and after sex. This practice is based on a theory that suggests peeing after sex can help flush out any bacteria from your urinary tract.

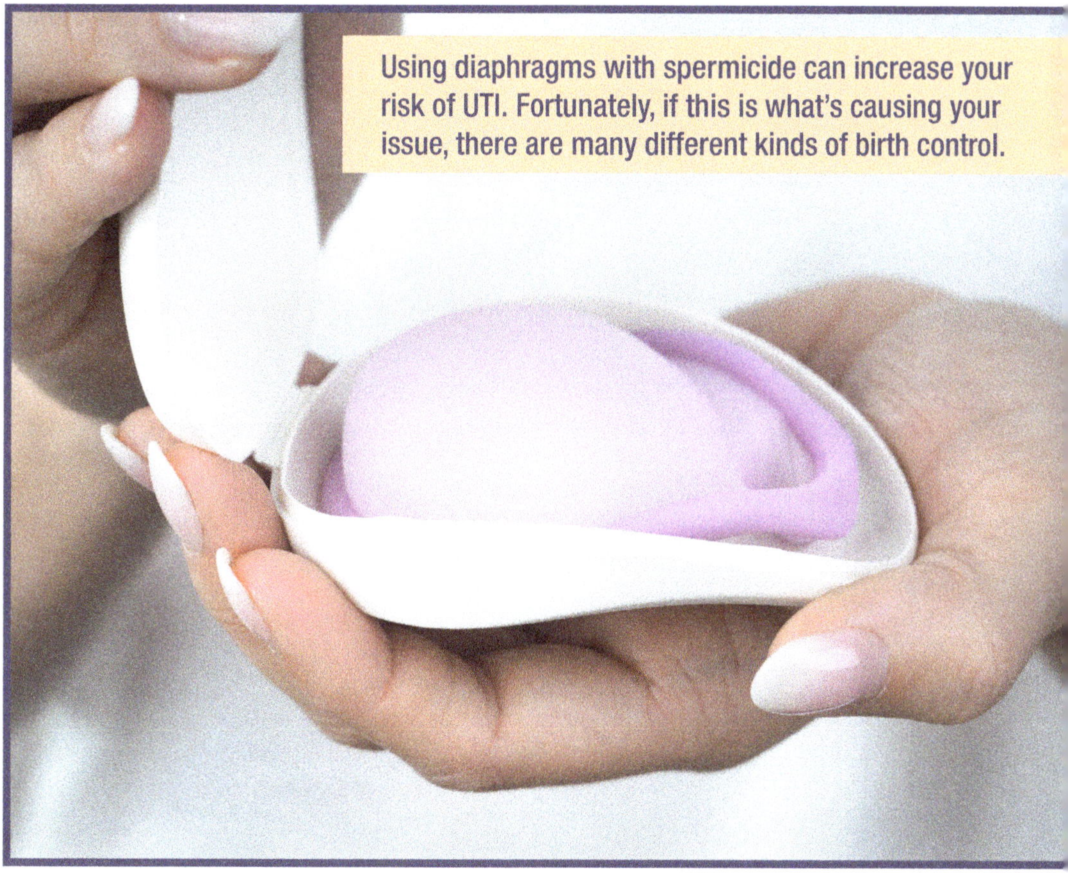

Using diaphragms with spermicide can increase your risk of UTI. Fortunately, if this is what's causing your issue, there are many different kinds of birth control.

AT GREATER RISK

Some people are at greater risk for UTIs than others. This includes people with spinal cord injuries, weakened immune systems, and diabetes. People in these at-risk groups might deal with frequent UTIs and have to be on the lookout for the symptoms before they worsen.

People who have spinal cord injuries (SPI) are at higher risk for UTIs than the general population. These injuries often require the person to use a catheter to urinate. A catheter is a thin tube that is inserted into the urethra. It allows urine to flow from the bladder into a drainage bag. The catheter can be another way that bacteria are introduced into the bladder. The catheter needs to be kept clean and replaced frequently to prevent a UTI.

People with abnormalities in their urinary tracts can often get more UTIs. For instance, some people develop pouches in their bladders called diverticula. A pouch like this allows urine to collect inside instead of being voided during urination. The stagnant urine is a breeding ground for bacteria. Other people have a ureter or urethra that is very narrow. This might prevent urine from leaving the kidney or bladder in the normal way. If urine stays too long in the urinary tract, an infection might develop.

Diabetes is a disease in which people have high levels of sugar, or glucose, in their blood. Type 1 diabetes occurs when the body doesn't produce enough insulin. Insulin is necessary to use and store the glucose that comes from food. People with type 2 diabetes don't respond well to the insulin their bodies

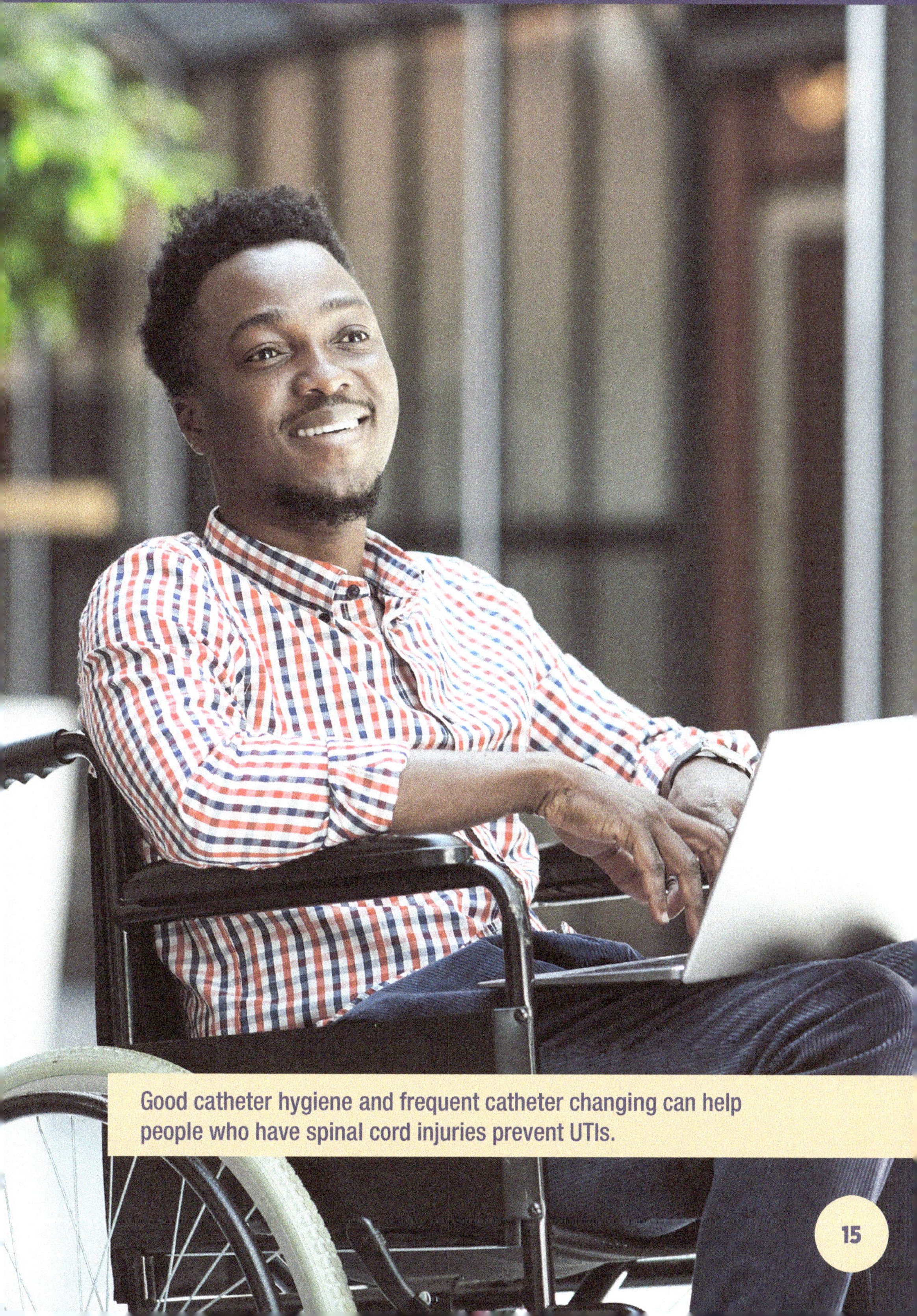

Good catheter hygiene and frequent catheter changing can help people who have spinal cord injuries prevent UTIs.

make. Diabetics get UTIs at a higher rate than the rest of the population. There are several reasons why. One reason is that people with diabetes have more glucose in their urine. The glucose provides food for the invading bacteria to multiply. Another reason is that some diabetics have nerve damage in their bladders. Their bladders don't contract enough to completely empty when they urinate. Urine left in the bladder for a long time provides an environment where bacteria can grow. A third reason is that diabetes can lead to reduced circulation of the blood. This reduces the ability of white blood cells, which fight infection, to get to the bacteria and kill it.

UTIs are also common in people whose immune systems are compromised by other conditions. Pregnant women are also susceptible because of hormonal changes in the body. A growing uterus can press on the bladder, preventing it from completely emptying. Transgender people who go through lower-body gender-affirming surgeries such as vaginoplasty (creating a vagina) and phalloplasty (creating a penis) may also have UTIs and other urologic issues. They should tell their doctors whenever they have UTIs or other urologic issues so they can quickly treat the infection and figure out what might be causing the problem.

MYTHS AND FACTS

MYTH
Getting a UTI means someone is sexually active.

FACT
There are many causes behind UTIs. Children, teens, and older adults can all suffer from UTIs. Sometimes they are caused by underlying health conditions, inadequate bathroom hygiene, or other circumstances.

MYTH
Male UTIs aren't as serious as female UTIs.

FACT
UTIs are more common in biologically female individuals. However, when biologically male individuals have UTIs, the infection is often more complicated and dangerous.

MYTH
UTIs will always clear up on their own.

FACT
Some minor UTIs may clear up on their own; however medical treatment is necessary in the case of complicated UTIs. It's important to seek medical advice as soon as you feel symptoms.

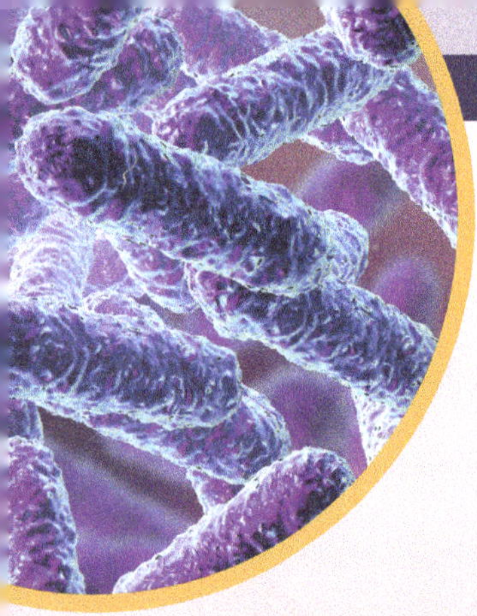

CHAPTER 2

DIFFERENT TREATMENTS FOR UTIS

If you're a teen who has just become sexually active, you might be nervous to tell anyone that you have a UTI. You might think your parents will be angry with you or disappointed in you. This kind of secrecy and shame has led many teens to suffer with a UTI without the right treatment.

It's important to know the signs and symptoms of a UTI. It's also important to reach out to a trusted adult—such as a school nurse or parent—to get treatment. If you're nervous to tell your parent about the fact that you had sex, you can just tell them you have a UTI so they can take you to a doctor. You may also be able to go to a school clinic or an outside clinic (which you may have to pay for) to get treatment. The most important thing is your health and well-being, and treatment is often necessary to get rid of a UTI.

SIGNS AND SYMPTOMS

Knowing the signs and symptoms of a UTI can help you spot it quickly and treat it before it becomes a major infection. When you have a UTI, one of the symptoms is the need to urinate frequently. However, even if you feel you have to pee, you may have difficulty passing the urine. Not only is this annoying, it can be painful. You might feel a burning sensation. Both the urge and burning sensation are caused by an inflamed and irritated bladder and urethra. This inflammation causes the muscles of the bladder to spasm, which produces the urge to pee. The urge and burning can vary in severity. Some people feel burning and pain all the time. Some report only a feeling of pressure.

You can also look to the color of your urine as a sign. Usually urine is light yellow. If yours is dark yellow, this may be an indication that you are dehydrated and need to drink more water. Cloudy urine is a symptom of a UTI. The cloudiness is caused by an abundance of white blood cells, which are there to fight infection. The infection may also cause blood to leak into the bladder. The blood may give your urine a pink tinge.

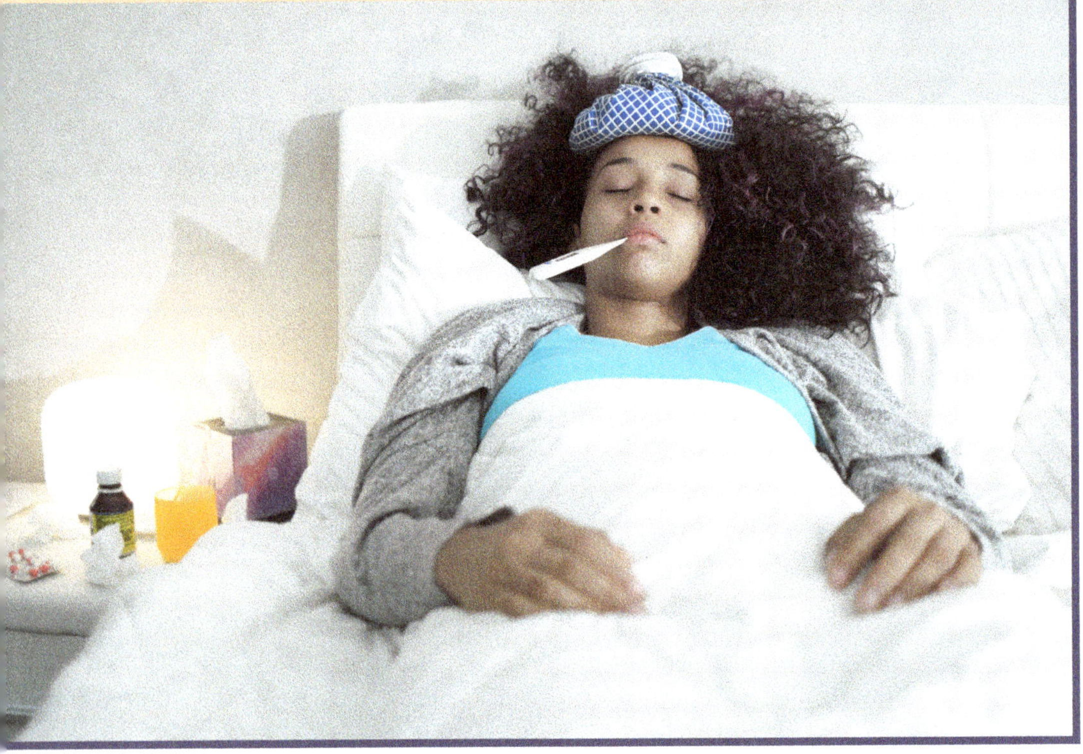

If you have a fever with your UTI, it's important to contact your doctor right away. A fever is a sign that you might have a bladder infection.

There may be other symptoms that point to a bladder infection. A body fighting an infection may result in a fever. Even a rise of a degree or two can slow bacteria's growth. Some people feel nausea, which may lead to vomiting. Fevers may make you shiver as if you're cold. Some people feel an ache in their lower abdomen. They might also feel tired and weak as their body tries to fight the infection. If you have a fever, nausea, or vomiting, it's a sign that you need to get treatment—fast.

THE FIRST STEP TO RELIEF

Life is busy—and no one has time for a UTI. In addition to school, you may have sports, clubs, a job, and homework. Even though you have a lot going on, you still need to make the time to see a health professional if you feel symptoms of a UTI. That's because an untreated UTI can turn into something more serious than a scheduling issue—a kidney infection. If you can't get into your doctor's office, you'll need to visit an urgent care center or hospital emergency room.

The first step at the doctor's office or clinic is to diagnose the UTI. You will be asked for a clean-catch urine specimen. The doctor or nurse will ask you to go into a bathroom and clean your genital area with an antiseptic disposable wipe. Then you need to pee into a sterile cup. Your urine will be tested to look for white

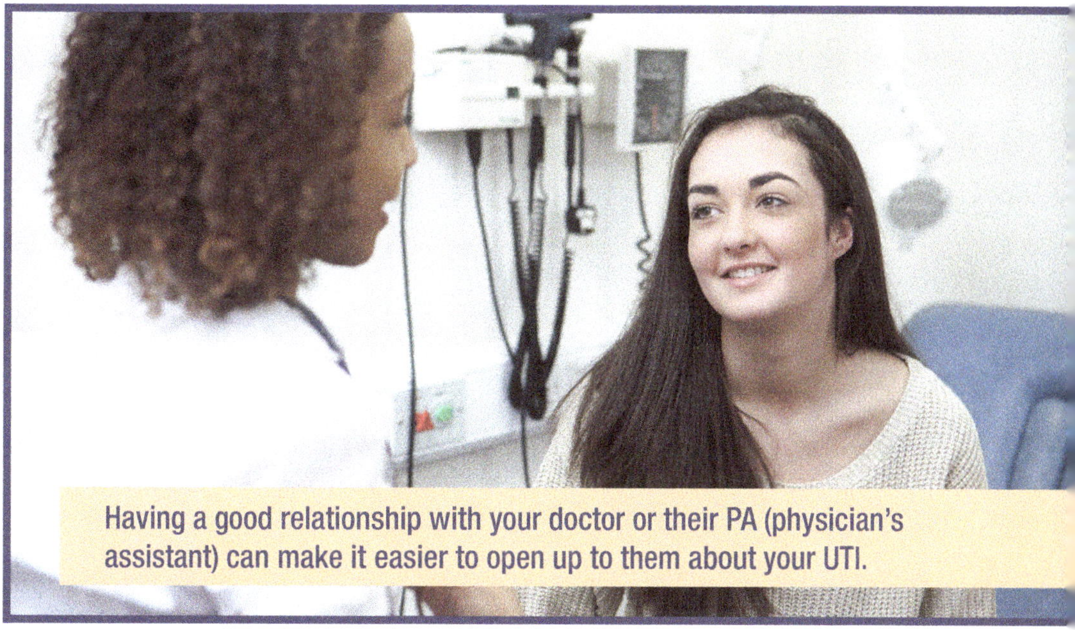

Having a good relationship with your doctor or their PA (physician's assistant) can make it easier to open up to them about your UTI.

blood cells, red blood cells, and bacteria. If any of these are present, the doctor will prescribe an antibiotic. You will need to fill the prescription at a pharmacy as soon as possible.

Once you start taking the antibiotic, a series of pills taken several times a day, you should start feeling better. Some patients will be given a three- to five-day course of antibiotics. Others might need to take the pills for seven to ten days. You need to take every pill, even if you start feeling better before the pills run out. You need to completely kill off the bacteria or the infection will come back. If you are feeling a lot of pain, the doctor can prescribe a medication to relieve the muscle spasms and pain in your bladder. This medication will turn your urine a bright orange color. It will usually make you feel more comfortable within a few hours. If after a few days you are not feeling better, you need to call your doctor and ask them what to do. They might want you to come back to see what's going on and make sure there are no issues with their recommended treatment.

CARING FOR YOURSELF

So, you've gotten a UTI diagnosis from a doctor and you've started taking the prescribed antibiotics. What other steps can you do to feel better? First, most medical professionals suggest that you drink a lot of water to flush out the bacteria. You need to allow your body to rest. It's a good idea to stop playing sports and engaging in any intense exercise for a few days. Sleep allows your body to recover. Since you are not contagious, you don't need to stay home from school unless you are in too much pain to concentrate or are going to the bathroom too much.

Make sure to eat a healthy diet while treating your UTI. There are some drinks that may irritate your bladder and cause pain with urination. Avoid coffee, alcohol, and soft drinks that contain citrus juices and caffeine. A warm heating pad on your abdomen will make you feel better. Make a follow-up visit to the doctor if you don't start feeling better within three or four days.

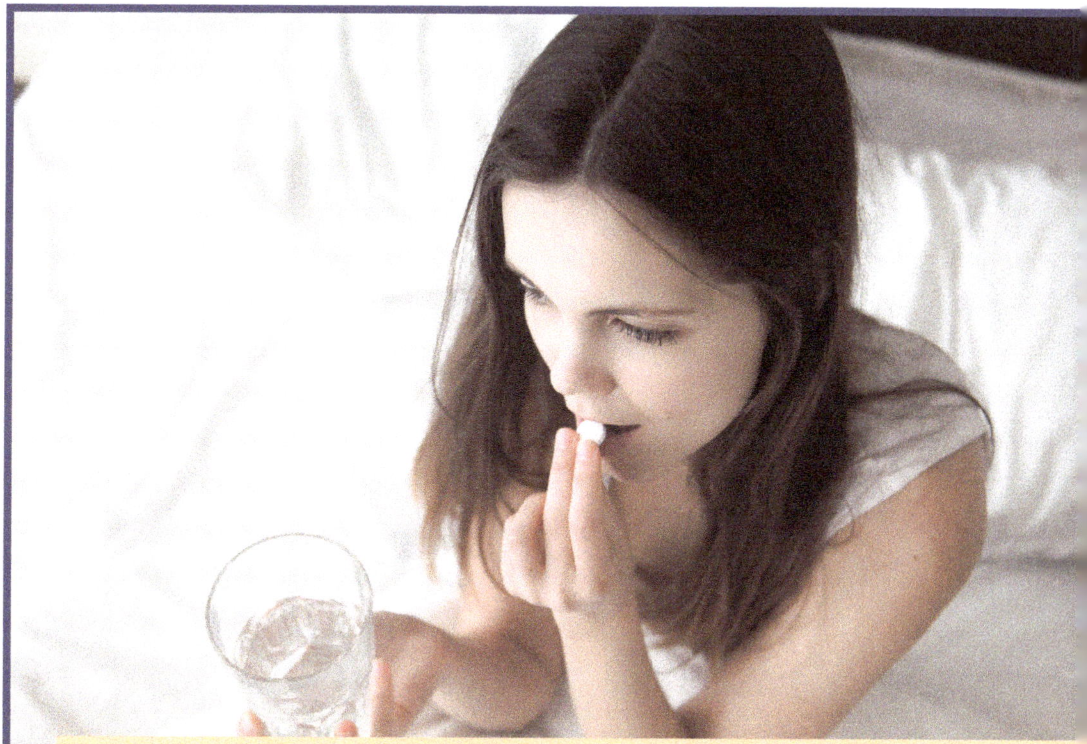

Doctors give very specific instructions for using antibiotics. Make sure to follow them. You can set an alarm in your phone to remind you to take your antibiotic at the right time.

ANTIBIOTICS: THE GOOD AND THE BAD

Antibiotics can be life-saving medicines. Since 1928, antibiotics have helped cure infections such as pneumonia, tuberculosis, and whooping cough. This saves many lives each year, so antibiotics are prescribed often. For most UTIs, antibiotics are the key to treatment and ultimately, relief.

But doctors are now concerned that if antibiotics are overused, there is a risk that some bacteria will become resistant, meaning the antibiotic becomes less effective against a particular type of bacterium. That's why it's important to only take antibiotics if a doctor has prescribed them to you for a specific issue.

Antibiotics also sometimes have side effects, such as a yeast infection. Antibiotics, by killing off bacteria, change the normal pH, or acidity level, in the vagina. A yeast infection is caused by a fungus called candida. Candida lives in the vagina in small amounts. When the pH changes, the yeast can grow and multiply. Symptoms of a yeast infection include vaginal itching and irritation and a cottage cheese–like discharge. Yeast infections can be treated by antifungal creams, ointments, tablets, or suppositories. The medications are available over the counter at most pharmacies. If the treatment doesn't clear up the infection, you need to let your doctor know. Some people claim that eating yogurt or taking probiotics prevents yeast infections while they are on antibiotics. While antibiotics have side effects, they are often more manageable than the complications that come from a severe UTI.

While most often not serious, UTIs can be a major disruption as they cause people to lose work and school time. Antibiotics have proven to be a quick, safe, and effective treatment for patients who use them correctly. UTI sufferers need to follow their doctors' instructions. Proper treatment and lots of rest and hydration can get you back on your feet in a few days.

Some antibiotics may make you drowsy, or overly tired. It's important to take time to sleep as much as your body needs.

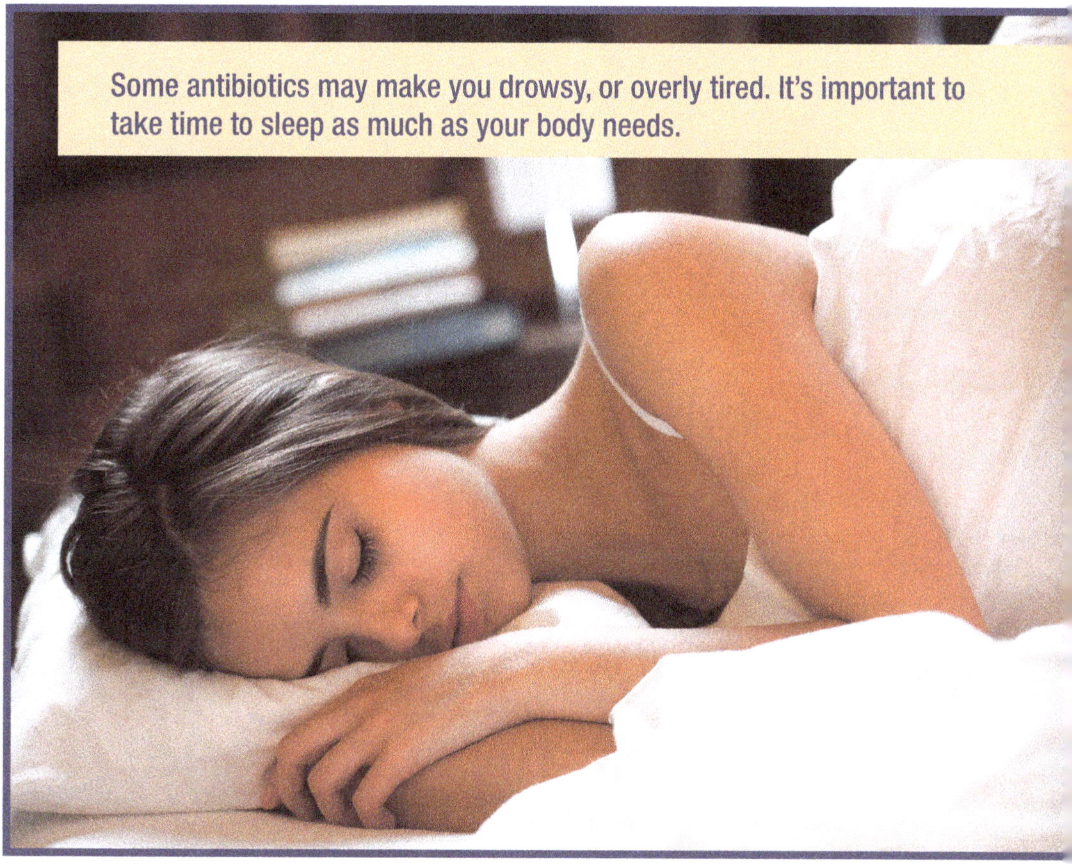

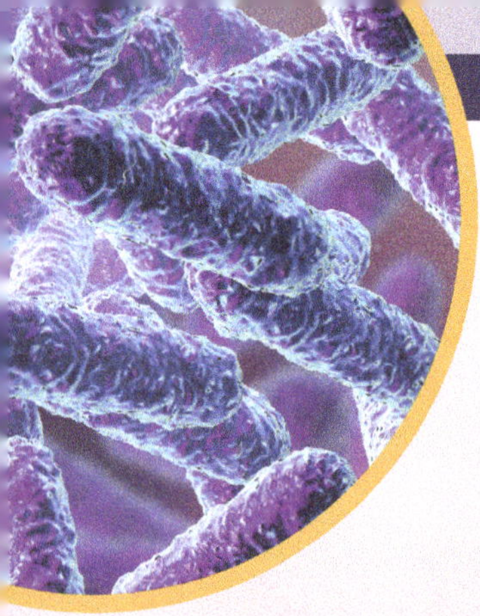

CHAPTER 3

UTI PREVENTION

Thanks to antibiotics, doctors have more ways to treat UTIs than ever. But you'll still want to avoid infection whenever possible. For some people, UTIs might be hard to prevent because of underlying health issues. Other people, however, can work to prevent UTIs from happening through hygiene practices, nutrition, hydration, and taking care of their sexual health.

HYGIENE HYPE

You probably know some basic hygiene practices, like showering often, brushing your teeth, and washing your hands. Hygiene practices help you stay clean and healthy to prevent illness and infection. We learn hygiene from parents and teachers when we're younger. As you hit puberty, you may also learn how to prevent illness and infection in health class and physical education (PE).

However, sometimes parents and teachers don't discuss bathroom procedures after you're potty trained or discuss sex as you hit puberty. These topics can be seen as inappropriate. However, it's very important to know about bathroom and sexual hygiene to prevent UTIs. Teens most often learn how to prevent UTIs after they have had one. But educating yourself before a UTI hits can help save you the trouble of going through one.

If you're a biologically female person, the most effective way to avoid getting a UTI is to prevent bacteria from getting near your vagina and urethra. Proper wiping from the front of the genital area to back is essential, as bacteria from the anus can cause UTIs. People who menstruate need to replace tampons and pads often, at least every couple of hours, to avoid a buildup of bacteria. Doctors recommend that you drink a lot of water to flush any bacteria out of your bladder. The most common way of measuring if you are drinking enough is that your urine stays a pale yellow color. If it's dark yellow, you aren't drinking enough water and need to hydrate.

Going to the bathroom often is an important strategy for preventing UTIs. There are many reasons why some people wait to urinate. They may be working hard on a project. The bathroom may be in an inconvenient location. Students may be discouraged from asking for a restroom pass because it's a distraction in class. You may find yourself trying to hold your urine because you

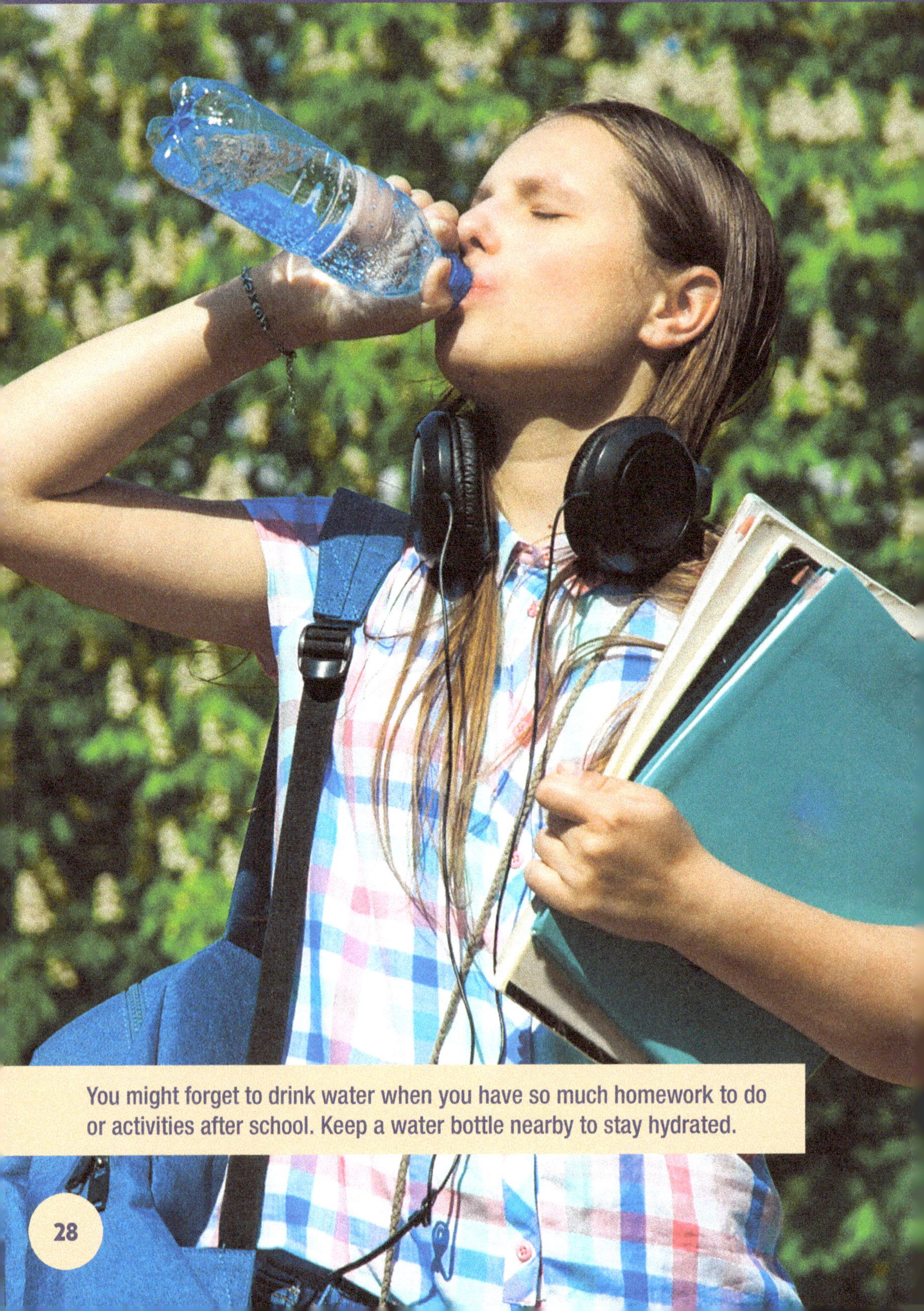

You might forget to drink water when you have so much homework to do or activities after school. Keep a water bottle nearby to stay hydrated.

don't want to interrupt a movie, miss a play in a game, or wait in a long restroom line. The longer the urine is in your bladder, the easier it is for bacteria to multiply. Health professionals encourage everyone to empty their bladders at least every few hours. If you're drinking as much water as you should be, you should be ready to visit the restroom that often.

You may enjoy soaking in a bubble bath as a way of relaxing tired and tense muscles at the end of a long day. But doctors encourage biologically female individuals, especially those prone to UTIs, to shower instead of taking baths. They should at least avoid the soap or bath salts used to produce the bubbles and fragrance in a bath. Substances in the bubble mixture can irritate the urethra. This irritation can cause a burning sensation during urination. This pain may cause you to avoid going to the bathroom. The pain might also cause you to not wipe completely.

The kind of underwear people wear can also make a difference in preventing UTIs. Nylon underwear traps moisture near the body, especially when it's hot outside. Bacteria love to grow in warm, moist places. To prevent UTIs, doctors advise wearing cotton underwear instead. Many people think they are safe with just a small strip of cotton in their underwear near the genitals. However, any fabric that is nonbreathable near the vagina or urethra will trap moisture. Thongs also put people at increased risk, regardless of the fabric. The skinny shape leaves the vulva more exposed to whatever they are wearing, such as Lycra or spandex leggings. The thin band tends to move around, possibly transferring bacteria from one spot to another. Bikini underwear is a better choice for women who like a minimal look.

It may feel inconvenient to ditch the underwear you like or the bubble baths that calm you down. It may also feel inconvenient to stop what you're doing and pee every few hours. But doing these things can make a big difference in preventing UTIs.

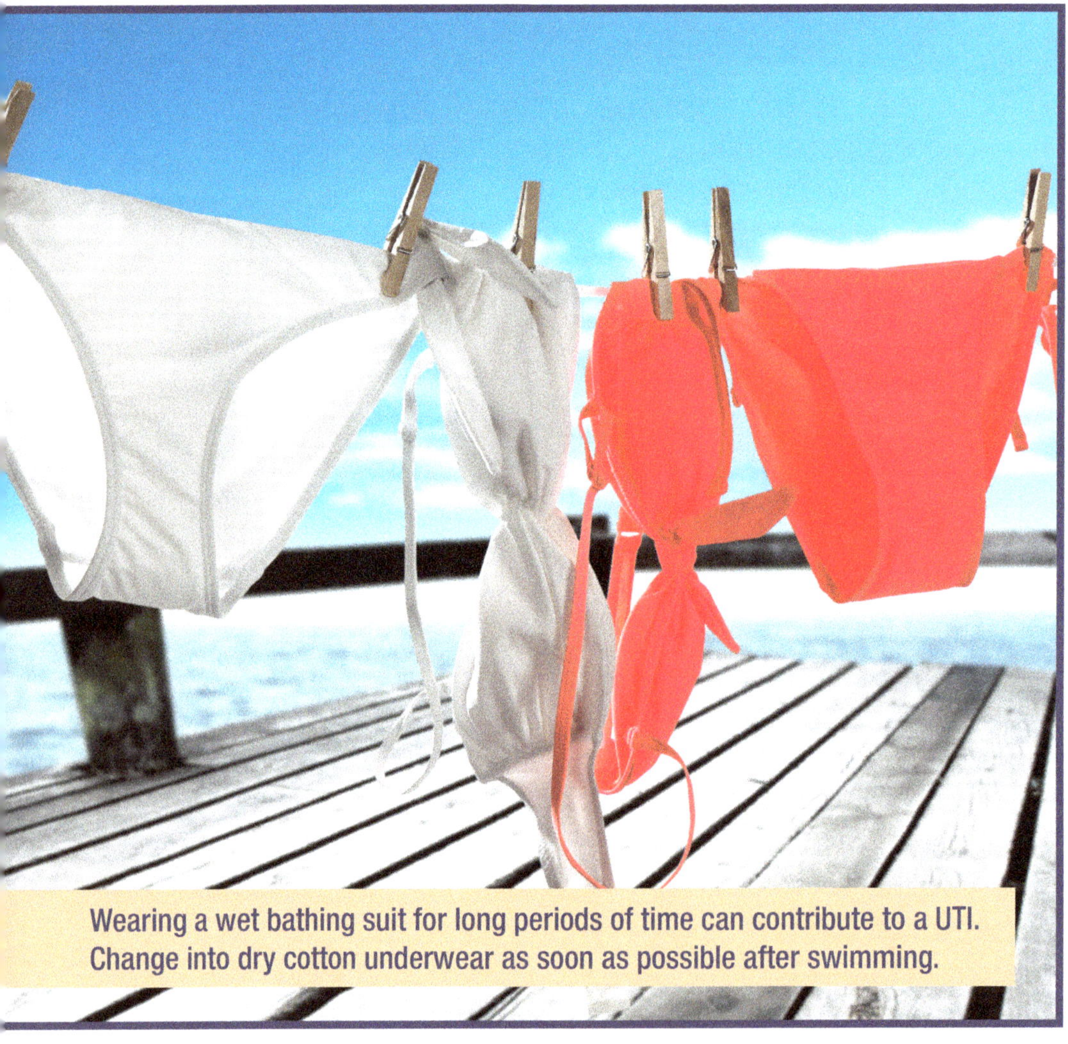

Wearing a wet bathing suit for long periods of time can contribute to a UTI. Change into dry cotton underwear as soon as possible after swimming.

THE DEAL WITH DOUCHING

The mid-20th century saw the start of a hygiene practice that we now know can lead to UTIs—douching. Douching is cleansing the vagina by squirting a solution of water, deodorizing chemicals, and soap into the vagina. At the time, many people thought this was just a part of good hygiene practices. Medical professionals then found that this practice can upset the natural balance of the vagina. The vagina has a natural balance of bacteria and a natural pH (or acidity), and it's important to maintain it. Healthy vaginas have natural processes that keep them clean and natural odor is normal. Douche solutions kill off beneficial bacteria, allowing bad bacteria, such as *E. coli*, to grow. The bad bacteria can easily be pushed into the urethra, causing a UTI. Sprays used to deodorize the vaginal area can cause irritation. If a person wants to keep their vaginal area clean, they can use mild soaps and body washes with their daily shower.

NUTRITION MAKES A DIFFERENCE

When you're busy with school and other activities, sometimes what you eat doesn't seem that important. Packaged snacks are easy to grab and fill your stomach. But nutrition is one way to keep one's body working smoothly. Nutrients from food can boost a person's immune system and help them fight off infection and illness. Many doctors and nutritionists suggest eating five servings of fruits and vegetables a day. Eating many different fruits and vegetables in different colors—like mixed greens, red peppers, carrots, blueberries, and bananas—is good for your health. Whole-wheat grains and sources of lean protein are also very important. Yogurt with probiotics may help keep UTIs at bay as well. A 2020 study found that vegetarian diets may lower the risk of UTIs. Other foods you might avoid if you're prone to UTIs are artificial sweeteners, coffee, alcohol, and spicy foods because they can irritate the bladder. Rest and exercise are also important to maintaining one's health.

Some people struggling with recurrent UTIs swear by consuming cranberries to prevent new infections. For many years, people have used cranberry juice to help prevent UTIs. Cranberries contain a type of acid that seems to prevent bacteria from attaching to the urethra. Cranberries are very tart, so sugar is added

Eating nutritious foods and relaxing can help you recover faster from UTIs and other illnesses.

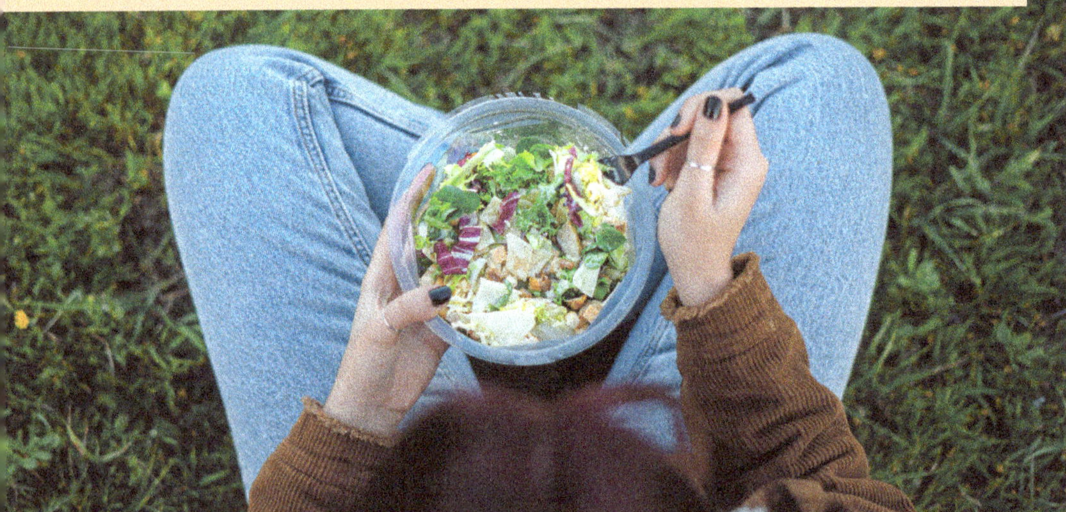

to most commercial cranberry juice. Sugar, however, is not helpful for people with UTIs. If you want to drink cranberry juice to prevent UTIs, drink it unsweetened or look for cranberry supplements in tablet form. Cranberry juice cannot cure a UTI, though, and some studies have shown that it may not be as effective as people believe.

SEX AND UTI PREVENTION

UTIs in teens and young adults are most often associated with sex. Frequent sex, certain birth control methods, and lack of proper sexual hygiene can increase the risk that you'll contract at UTI. But there are things you can do to help prevent UTIs. For example, if your birth control method might be causing your UTIs, you can discuss with your health care provider other forms of contraceptives you can use.

Your hygiene practices before, during, and after sex can also make a difference. Some doctors recommend certain urinary habits to reduce UTIs in sexually active women. Urinating before having sex reduces the amount of urine that can be infected by bacteria. Going to the bathroom right after having sex can flush out bacteria before it has a chance to establish itself in the urethra and bladder. It is also a good idea to clean hands and any sexual devices before sex, and clean your genital area with a mild soap and water after having sex. If you're using a lubricant, make sure it's water-soluble. If a person has frequent UTIs, their doctor may recommend a low dose of antibiotics to take after sex.

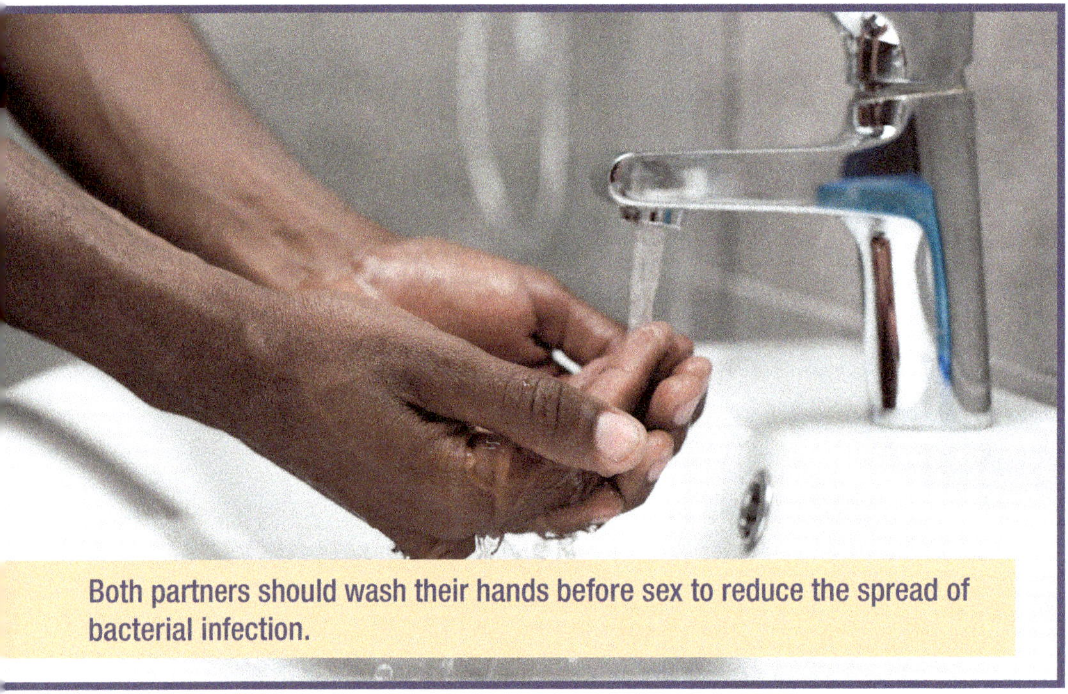

Both partners should wash their hands before sex to reduce the spread of bacterial infection.

THE FACTS ON FREQUENT UTIS

Getting one or two UTIs every year is normal for some people, especially biologically female people. However, if you get more than two UTIs a year, your doctor may consider your UTIs to be recurrent or frequent, which means they will want to figure out why it's happening and how to best treat you. First, your doctor may determine exactly which antibiotic to prescribe. One way to do this is to culture your urine. Usually to diagnose a UTI, a doctor or nurse will dip a stick into your urine to detect nitrates or white blood cells, which signal a UTI. A culture is done by putting some of your urine into a dish with a substance that encourages any bacteria to grow. Then the bacteria can be identified and a specific antibiotic prescribed. You might be asked to take the antibiotic for longer than a week.

Your health-care provider might want to see if your urinary tract is normal. There are several tests that can be done. One is a kidney and bladder ultrasound. A radiology technician will use a device called a transducer to bounce painless sound waves off your organs to create an image of their structure. This procedure is done in the doctor's office or an outpatient center. The images can show abnormalities in the organs and give your doctor a better idea of the issue.

A voiding cystourethrogram is an x-ray image of your bladder and urethra taken while your bladder is full. Your bladder will be filled with a special dye to make your organs clearly visible on the x-ray. Then you'll be

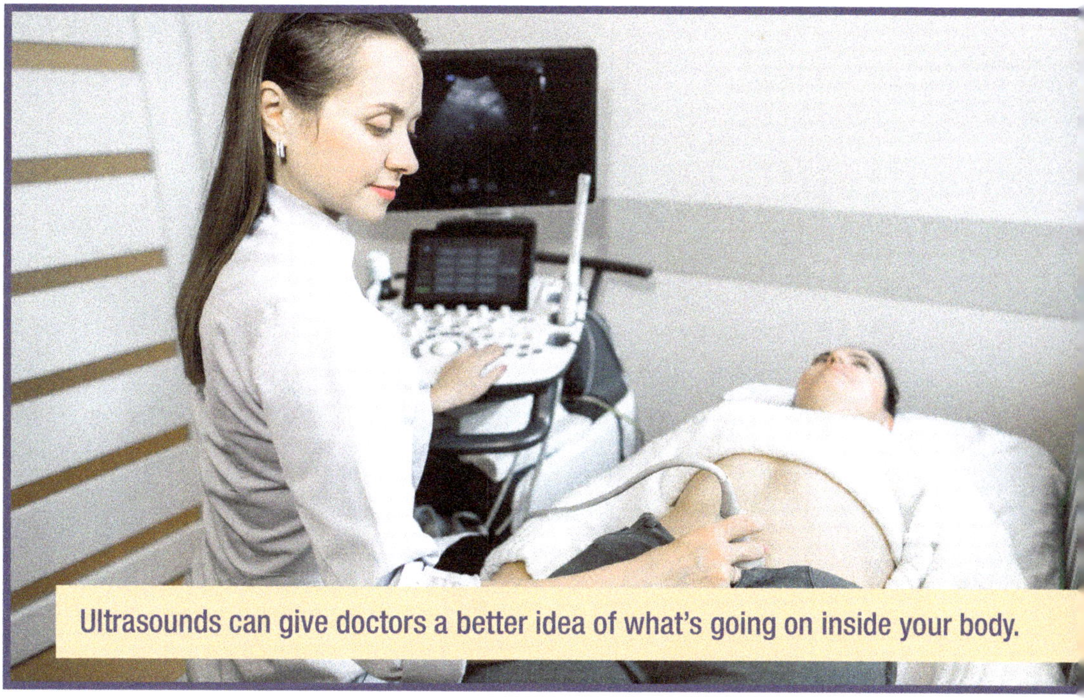

Ultrasounds can give doctors a better idea of what's going on inside your body.

asked to urinate into a container. The radiologist can see how your bladder works and if the flow of urine is normal.

Other tests that might be done are computerized tomography (CT) scans, magnetic resonance imaging (MRI), radionuclide scans, and urodynamics testing. These tests can find abnormalities and other problems that might provide reasons for your UTIs. You might be referred to a urologist, a doctor who specializes in diseases and conditions of the urinary tract. While medication cures most urinary tract infections, you might need surgery to correct a condition that may continue to give you UTIs. For instance, surgery might be necessary if there is tissue that obstructs the urethra.

For some patients who get recurrent UTIs, a doctor might prescribe antibiotics as UTI prevention as well as treatment. For instance, a person might take a one-dose antibiotic after having sex. Some people might be prescribed a continual low dose of antibiotics as a way of preventing UTIs. These therapies have side effects. Some might develop resistance to particular antibiotics if they take them for long periods of time. Others might develop yeast infections.

Most people who get a UTI will learn the strategies that are effective in preventing them. People who have recurrent UTIs will have to work with their health-care providers to find the right antibiotic for their particular strain of bacteria, as well as helpful nutritional and behavioral practices to keep UTIs away.

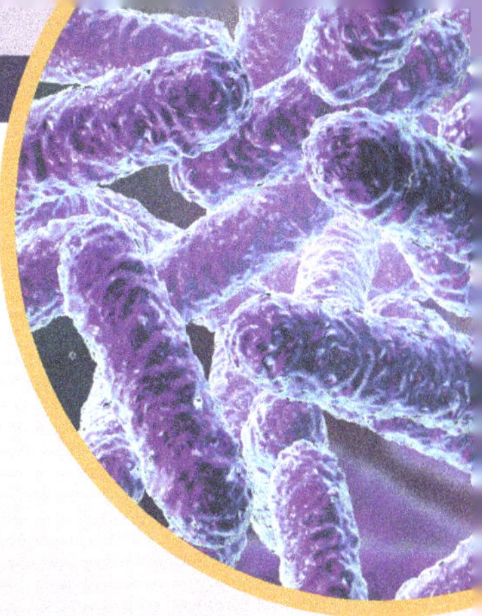

CHAPTER 4

UTI RISKS AND COMPLICATIONS

UTIs are nothing new. Ancient peoples had them too, though they didn't have antibiotics to help. An ancient Egyptian papyrus, or scroll, recommended herbal treatments for urinary problems. The Greek physician Hippocrates thought that urinary pain was caused by disharmony in the body. Roman and Arab physicians expanded knowledge about urinary issues.

It wasn't until the 19th century that people discovered that microorganisms caused disease. This discovery sparked more advances in the treatment of UTIs in the 20th century. Luckily, doctors are now better able to diagnose and treat UTIs than ever. Over-the-counter home self-test kits are available to diagnose your own UTIs. There have been huge advances in imaging technology, such as x-rays, ultrasounds, nuclear imaging, and MRIs. New antibiotics have been developed that are safer and more effective than older medications. Physicians are finding ways to more accurately match a person's particular strain of bacteria with an antibiotic that specifically targets it. Researchers are experimenting with vaccines in the form of nasal sprays to prevent UTIs.

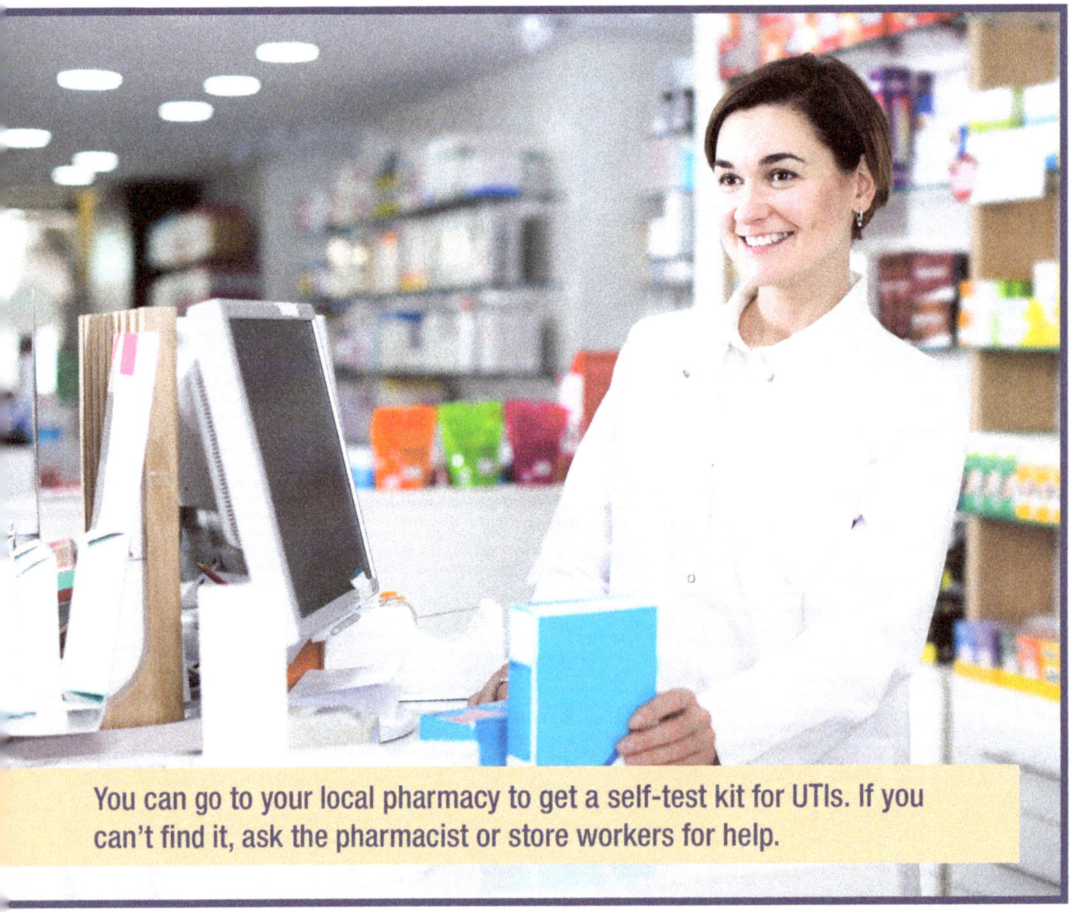

You can go to your local pharmacy to get a self-test kit for UTIs. If you can't find it, ask the pharmacist or store workers for help.

Many people are able to recover quickly from a UTI with antibiotics and a doctor's care. But even in this age of UTI treatments, risks and complications are still an issue. Older people, people with diabetes, and people with kidney issues may even develop a possibly fatal condition called sepsis. Around 13,000 people die from UTI complications each year in the United States.

WHEN UTIS TURN SERIOUS

Most people with UTIs experience no serious complications, especially if they get to a doctor quickly after symptoms arise. However, some infections turn serious, especially for certain populations. Complications are more likely in people with preexisting health conditions, such as diabetes or a weakened immune system. Pregnant women sometimes develop complications if a UTI is left untreated. These complications could include preterm labor and low birth weight in their baby. Even if you don't have a preexisting condition, if you don't get better when the doctor predicted, you need to make a follow-up appointment.

Although males have UTIs less frequently, those being treated for a UTI are at risk for complications that affect the prostate. The prostate is a walnut-sized gland that secretes the fluid that makes up semen. A UTI can spread infection to the prostate, causing prostatitis. This condition can be treated by antibiotics. If the issue is severe, a biologically male person suffering from a UTI might call a specialist doctor called a urologist. Urologists specialize in diseases of the urinary tract and male reproductive organs.

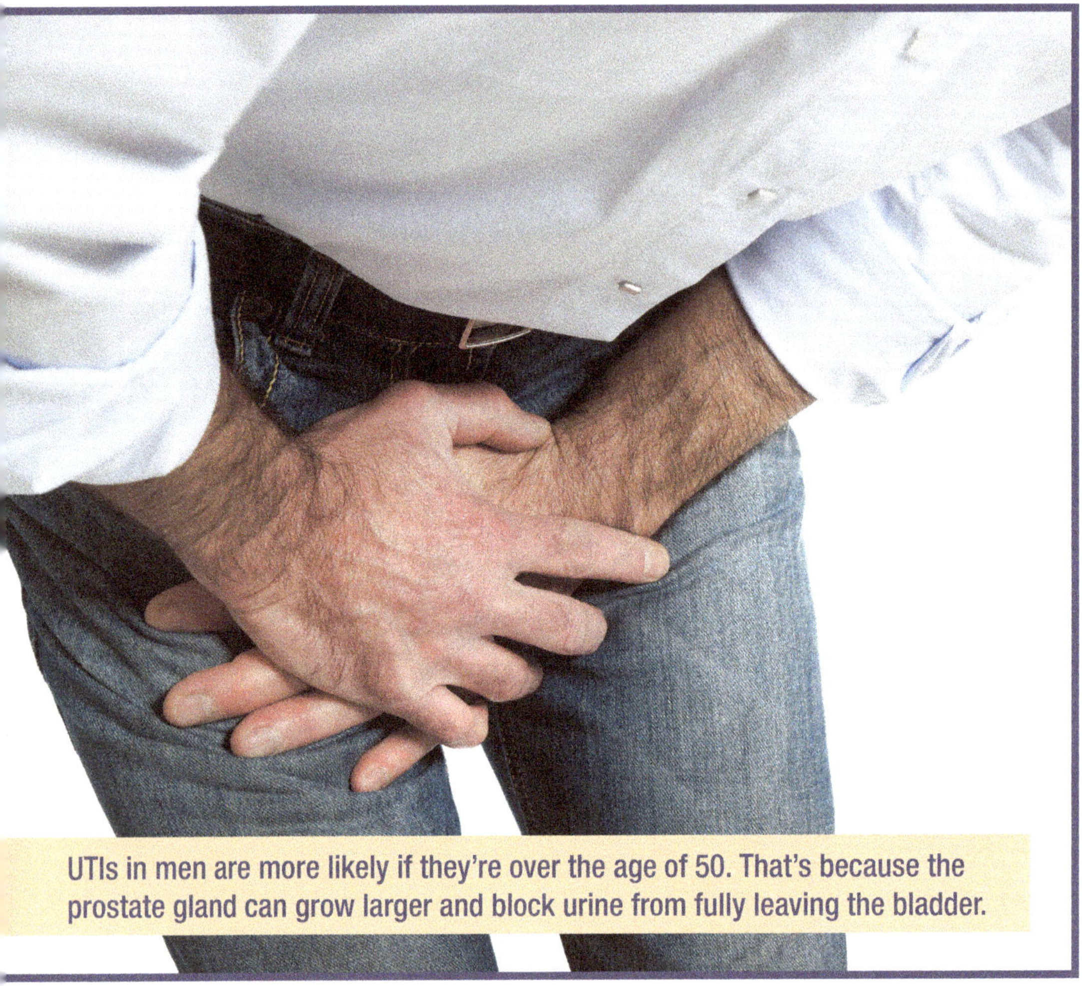

UTIs in men are more likely if they're over the age of 50. That's because the prostate gland can grow larger and block urine from fully leaving the bladder.

Because the kidneys are near the bladder, bacteria can travel from the bladder to the kidneys. The symptoms of a kidney infection develop quickly. You might feel pain in your side, in your lower back, and around your genitals. You may develop a fever and chills. You will generally feel tired, weak, and sick. You will probably lose your appetite and may develop diarrhea.

DOCTOR'S ORDERS

To prevent complications from a UTI or kidney infection, it's important to follow your doctor's instructions. If you develop a kidney infection, your doctor will most likely prescribe more antibiotics and then schedule a follow-up visit in about two weeks. This is the length of time for a kidney infection to be resolved. As with a UTI, getting a lot of rest and drinking a lot of fluids will help you feel better.

It's also important to be responsible about your antibiotic use. The Centers for Disease Control and Prevention (CDC), recommends you use antibiotics only when they are likely to be beneficial. While antibiotics are beneficial for certain bacterial infections like UTIs and strep throat, they shouldn't be taken for viral infections like colds or flus. The CDC also recommends that you follow your doctor's instructions exactly. Don't stop taking the pills before you run out, even if you are feeling better. If you stop too soon, some bacteria may survive. Don't take antibiotics prescribed for someone else or those that have been prescribed for another illness. Don't share your antibiotics with someone else. By using antibiotics as they're intended, you can get better faster and work against antibiotic resistance.

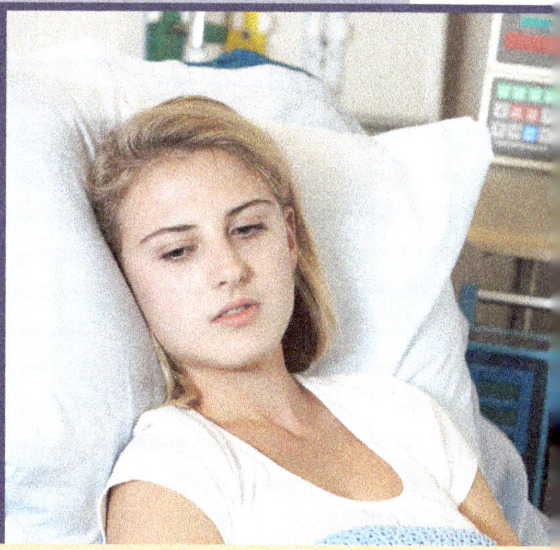

Some UTIs require hospitalization. This allows doctors to give patients the medicine and fluids they need and keep track of how they're doing.

Very rarely, a UTI can be the source of a life-threatening illness. Some bacteria are hard to get rid of because they've become resistant to most common antibiotics. A kidney infection that's resistant to antibiotics can lead to sepsis. Bacteria get into the blood, which triggers the immune system to release chemicals into the blood. The inflammation that results from these chemicals can lead to organ failure. This is what happened to a 20-year-old Brazilian model. In 2009, Mariana Bridi contracted a UTI that was resistant to antibiotics. The illness progressed to a kidney infection and then to sepsis. Eventually she died from complications of the infection. In 2021, fans were stunned when it was revealed that 65-year-old actress Tanya Roberts (who acted in *Charlie's Angels* and *That '70s Show*) died from a UTI that had developed into sepsis.

WHAT IS ANTIBIOTIC RESISTANCE?

Bacteria are so small we need a microscope to see them. They also inhabit every environment on Earth—from deserts to the deep sea to our urinary tract. But some bacteria strains are also some of the deadliest organisms on Earth. We use antibiotics to treat bacterial infections, and that's greatly reduced illness and death from infectious diseases. However, bacteria are great at adapting to challenges; since the drugs have been used so widely, some bacteria have adapted to the antibiotics. These adaptations reduce or eliminate the effectiveness of the drugs that are made to cure the diseases. According to a 2019 CDC report, more than

2.8 million people in the United States become infected with bacteria that are resistant to antibiotics. More than 35,000 people die each year from these infections in the United States. Many more die from other conditions that were complicated by an antibiotic-resistant infection, such as pneumonia, sexually transmitted diseases, and skin diseases.

The United States isn't the only country that's battling this problem. Antibiotic resistance occurs everywhere in the world. The CDC calls it one of the world's most pressing public health problems. The effects are devastating. People who have infections caused by drug-resistant bacteria are likely to have longer and more expensive hospital stays. When the drug that is treating their infection doesn't work, patients require treatment with drugs that may be less effective, more toxic, and more expensive. These patients may suffer more and pay more for treatment. The patients also may spread their disease to family members, friends, and coworkers.

There are many causes of antibiotic resistance. One is the routine use of antibiotics in food-producing animals such as poultry and cattle. The bacteria in the animals develop resistance. Consumers then pick up the bacteria either in the preparation or the eating of the animals. Another cause is the use of antibiotics to treat viral infections. Too many people demand antibiotics from their doctors when they have viral infections such as a cold. Antibiotics cannot stop or prevent an infection caused by a virus. The CDC is currently studying the impact of widespread use of antibacterial soaps and solutions. Antibacterial products are essential in health-care settings. However, there may be a link between the widespread use of these products and an increase in antibiotic resistance. Instead of using antibacterial soap in everyday life, the CDC recommends basic handwashing with regular soap and water. While the risk of bacterial infections is concerning, the possibility of antibiotic-resistant bacteria is also worrisome.

10 GREAT QUESTIONS
TO ASK YOUR DOCTOR

1. Do alternative remedies (not antibiotics) work to treat a UTI?
2. Do alternative remedies work to prevent a UTI?
3. When might I start to feel relief from my UTI?
4. Can I spread my UTI to my family on a shared toilet seat?
5. Can I transmit my UTI to my partner through sex?
6. What are the side effects of the antibiotics you're prescribing?
7. Will antibiotics make my birth control method less effective?
8. What can I take to prevent a yeast infection while taking antibiotics?
9. Am I at risk for any complications from this UTI?
10. What happens if the antibiotics you prescribe don't work?

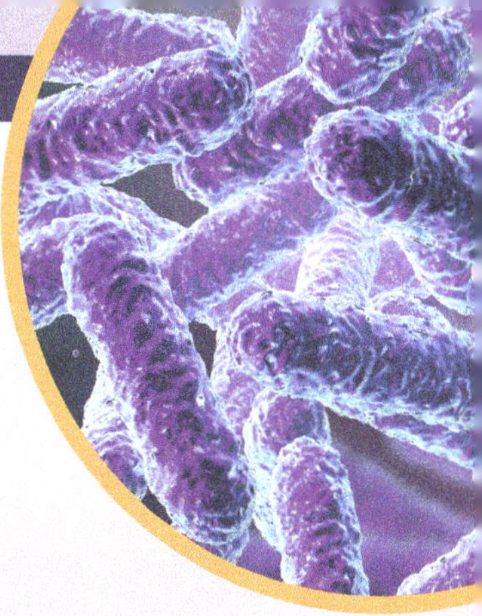

CHAPTER 5

DEALING WITH UTIS

Having a UTI can really put a damper on your plans. You likely have a lot of commitments between school, family, sports, friends, jobs, and volunteer work. Taking time off from those things to focus on recovering from a UTI can be upsetting. However, part of the process of becoming an adult is taking responsibility for your health. This means following your doctor's orders, learning as much as you can about your infection, taking advantage of resources that are available to you, and managing your emotional responses.

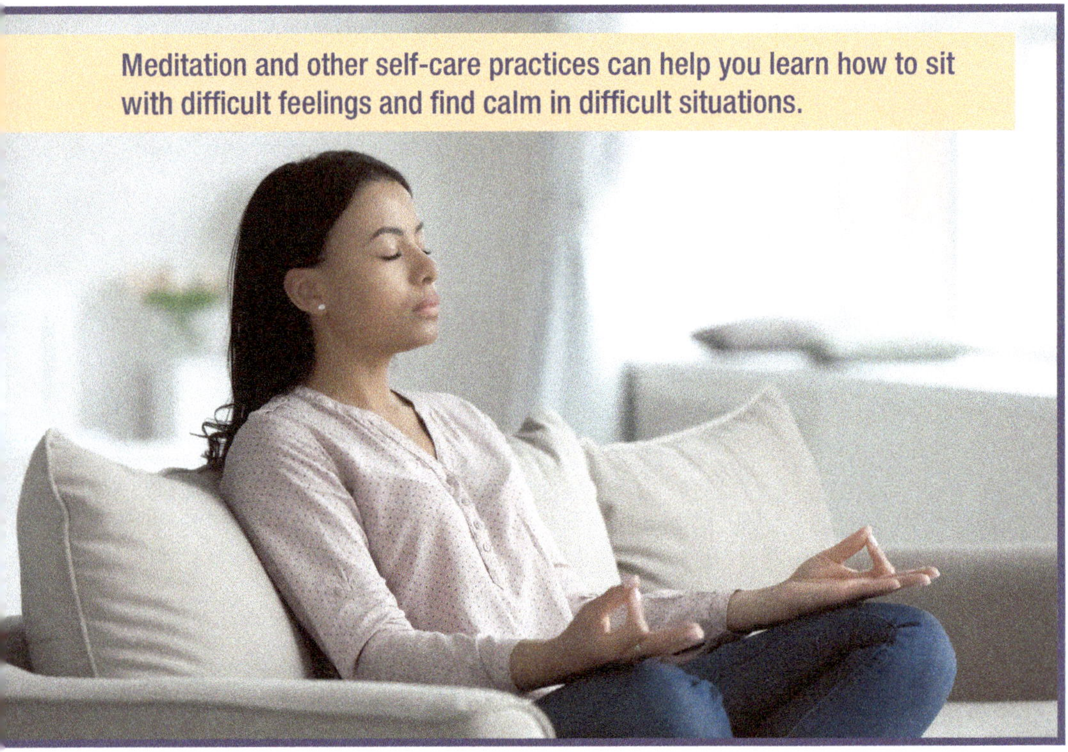

Meditation and other self-care practices can help you learn how to sit with difficult feelings and find calm in difficult situations.

As you care for your physical health, it's also important to check in with your mental well-being. Dealing with difficult emotions around your UTI can be a challenge. Learning more about your infection, as well as gathering coping tools, can help you feel more empowered as you deal with it.

DOS AND DON'TS

Listening to your doctor's instructions will give you a good sense of what to do or not do while you are recovering from your UTI. You were probably told to rest until you no longer have a fever and your temperature returns to normal. Resting gives your immune system a chance to fight the infection. A fever is a sign that white blood cells have arrived in your bladder to kill the bacteria. The body raises the heat level to stimulate the white blood cells and inhibit the growth of bacteria. A decreasing fever is a sign that the white blood cells have done their job. If you are taking antibiotics, it shouldn't take more than a day or two at home to start feeling a lot better.

When you do return to physical activity, you do need to take some precautions. If your clothing gets sweaty, change it immediately. Use the bathroom before and right after sports or PE classes. Drink a lot of water, more than usual. Do everything you can to minimize the chances that bacteria can get near your urethra.

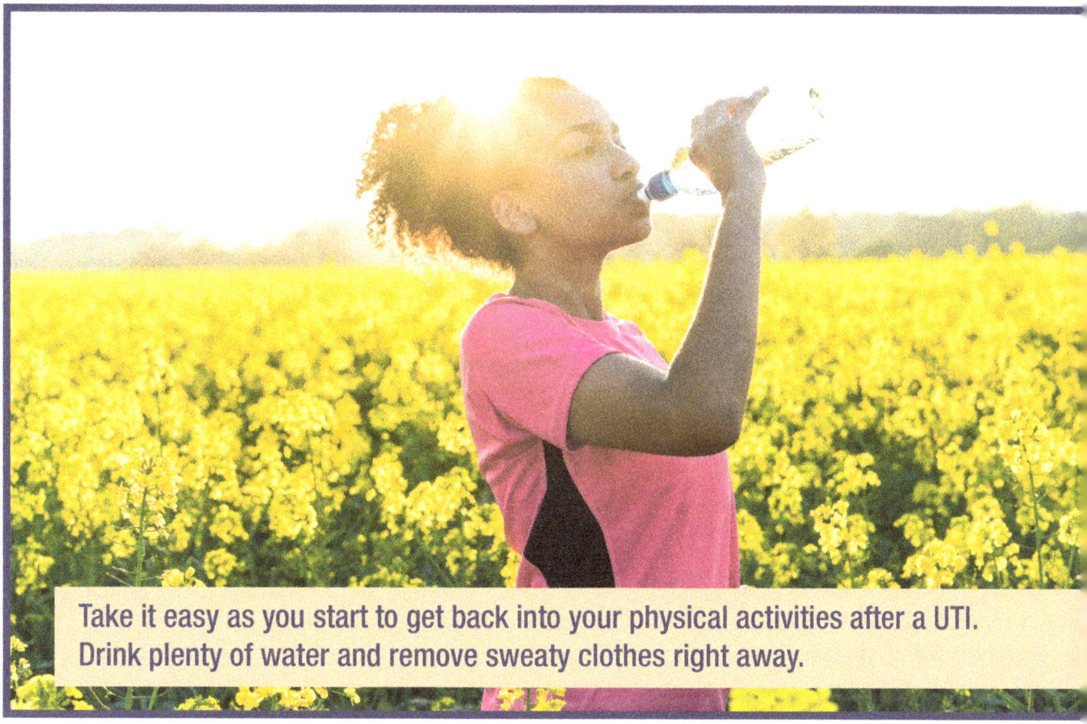

Take it easy as you start to get back into your physical activities after a UTI. Drink plenty of water and remove sweaty clothes right away.

Don't push yourself too much physically, especially if you still have a fever or weakness. It's also a good idea to not have sex while you're feeling sick. With time and patience, you'll start to feel better.

KNOWLEDGE IS POWER

The more you know, the more power you have. This is especially true when it comes to your health. You can access reliable health information at your doctor's office or family health clinic. Your health professionals may have informational handouts or brochures on UTIs that you can take home with you to read. They also may refer you to resources that will answer your questions.

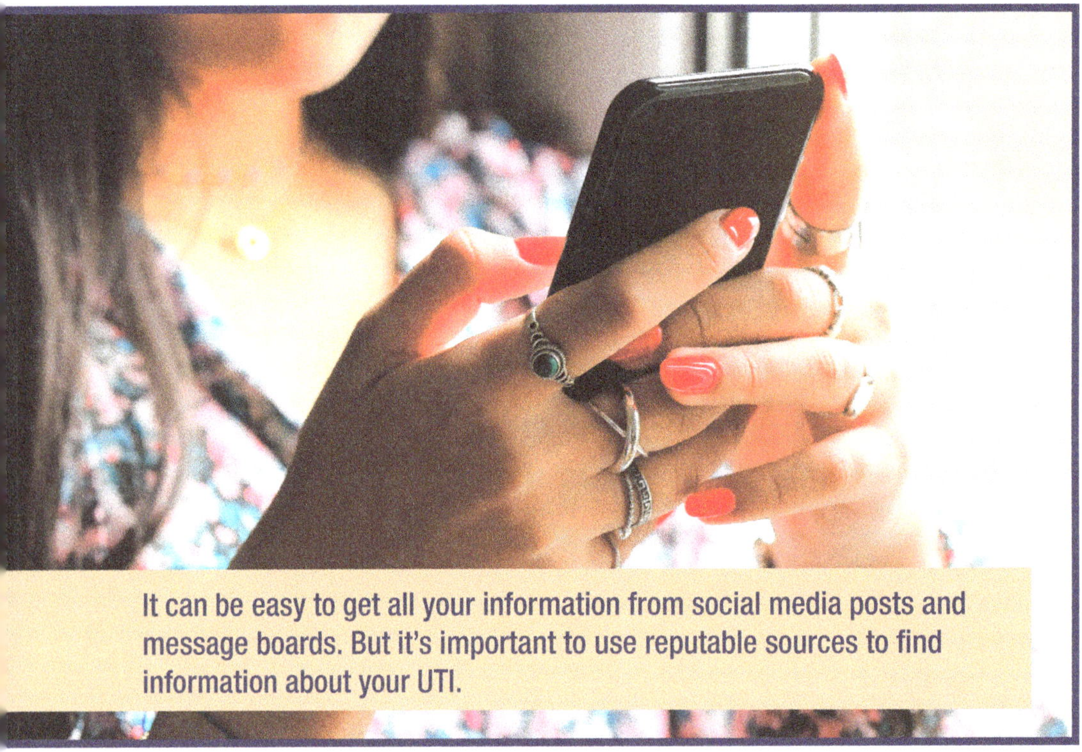

It can be easy to get all your information from social media posts and message boards. But it's important to use reputable sources to find information about your UTI.

Libraries are good places to find reference materials. Most public libraries have online databases that are available to anyone with a library card. The reference librarian at your local library branch can show you how to use these databases. Many schools provide databases for their students to use for research. All of these databases are likely to have current information on health topics.

One of the easiest places to find information is the internet. The challenge is to find websites with correct information. Steer clear of message boards, blogs, product reviews, or videos by anyone other than a real medical professional. Many people give advice for alternative products or treatments that have no basis in science. If you find articles written by doctors or nurses, you might find more accurate information. It's usually a good indication that a source is reputable if the website ends in .gov, .edu, or .org. Reputable hospitals may have trustworthy health and medical information available through their websites. One U.S. hospital that provides a wealth of research and resources is the Mayo Clinic. Through MayoClinic.com, thousands of physicians and researchers provide in-depth information on hundreds of diseases and conditions.

Disease-specific organizations offer websites dedicated to informing consumers about their particular disease. For instance, the National Institute of Diabetes and Digestive and Kidney Diseases has a well-organized website that offers great information about the symptoms, causes, and treatments of bladder infections.

GIVING SUPPORT AND EDUCATING OTHERS

Many people don't like to talk about UTIs. That can cause people suffering from UTIs to feel isolated or too nervous to seek help or support. It can be awkward to discuss a disease, especially one connected to taboo topics like urinating and sex. You may worry that your UTI will become a piece of gossip or something to be used against you. However, telling trusted people about your UTI can help you find emotional support and help as you recover.

What if your family and friends judge you for your UTI? If you have done your research and have accurate information at your fingertips, you can dispel any misconceptions family and friends may have about UTIs. From you, they can learn that the condition is not contagious, it is easily treated, and it sometimes, but not always, results from sexual activity. They can even cover for you if other people notice you disappearing to the restroom often.

If someone you know contracts a UTI, you can be a great support to them. Showing empathy for their pain and discomfort is usually appreciated. The sick person may be feeling embarrassed or guilty if they think they caused their own illness. If you know the facts about UTIs, you can help them realize that they have the power to prevent future UTIs. Encouraging them to rest, drink water, pay attention to nutrition, and take medicine regularly are all ways to show support.

If you have a UTI and are in an intimate relationship with someone, honest communication about your condition is essential. Your partner needs to know all the facts about what causes UTIs and how they can be prevented. They need to understand the connection between some forms of contraceptives and UTIs. Together you might need to research alternate forms of birth control. It will be uncomfortable to have sex while treating a UTI. It is a good idea to take a break from sexual activity while treating the condition. Supportive partners always care about your health and well-being above all else.

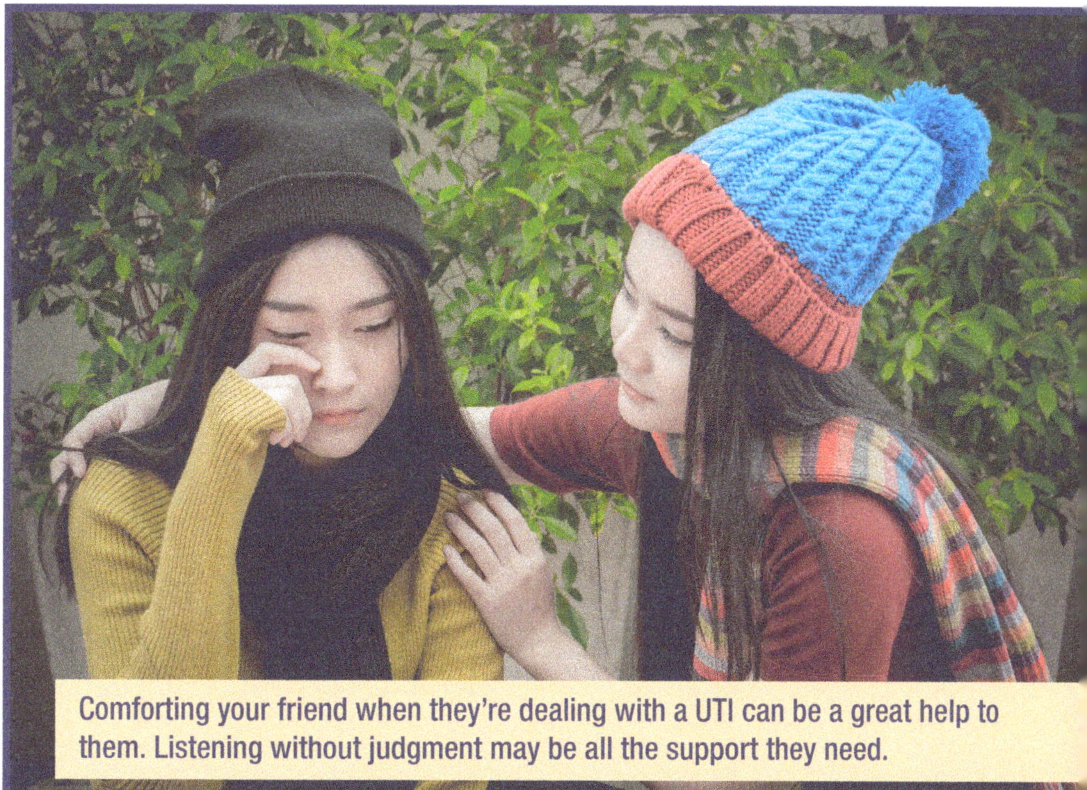

Comforting your friend when they're dealing with a UTI can be a great help to them. Listening without judgment may be all the support they need.

TO BE HONEST

You might worry about telling your friends, family, teachers, or sexual partner about your UTI. While it's good to share that information for support and help as you deal with your UTI, the most important person to tell is your doctor.

Pediatricians and family doctors can be your biggest allies in navigating through the health issues of adolescence and young adulthood. They have a lot of experience helping teens with questions about substance abuse, sexually transmitted diseases, and mental health issues. Even if you think they might judge you, remember that they've probably seen it all. But they need help from you. To accurately diagnose and treat an illness or condition, they need you to be completely honest. It may be difficult to admit that you are sexually active to a doctor who has been treating you since you were a baby. Your physician isn't there to judge you, just to help you get better. If you do feel uncomfortable with your doctor or feel judged, you may also be able to go to a clinic such as Planned Parenthood to get tested and treated for a UTI.

NOTIFYING THOSE WHO NEED TO KNOW

Maybe you've been in contact with your doctor, parents, and close friends about your UTI. Who else might need to know? As a teen, much of your day is spent at school. Attending classes and extracurricular activities will be difficult if you are having symptoms of a UTI, such as needing to go to the bathroom often and feeling pain in your pelvic area. Letting the appropriate people know about your UTI will make your day go more smoothly. Either you or a parent should first notify the school nurse that you are being treated for a UTI. They can work with you and your teachers to make sure your needs are met.

If your UTI is causing you significant symptoms, you or a parent may need to notify your teachers about your UTI. You most likely won't be attending school while your symptoms are at their worst and you still have a fever and pain. When you return to school, however, you still might have to get quickly to a restroom or go lie down for a few minutes. Supportive teachers who know about your UTI can issue a pass to the restroom or nurse's office without a lot of attention and embarrassment. After you return to school, you still might need a day or two of recovery before you participate in PE classes or sports. Make sure you keep your coaches in the loop. They shouldn't want you back to practice until you are completely recovered.

If you have a job, you can share with your manager that you have a UTI, but only if you feel very comfortable about doing so. You don't have to be specific with your boss. You may just say, "I'm not feeling well enough to work so I'm staying home today." Employers will not want you working if you're not at your best. You might need to bring an excuse from your doctor if you are out more than a day or two.

You might already have a counselor or mental health therapist for a separate issue, such as anxiety or depression. They can be a great resource for coping tools as you deal with your UTI if you share your diagnosis with them. If you don't already have mental health support, you can incorporate mental wellness tools such as breathing exercises, journaling, and meditation or reflection. Dealing with health issues is often easier when you're in a good headspace.

It may seem overwhelming to think of all the people who might need to know about your UTI. It's OK to only tell people on an as-needed basis to help you recover. Teachers, coaches, and school personnel will likely be sympathetic and nonjudgmental. They will want you to focus on recovery. As always, your health is the most important priority.

RESPONSIBILITY FOR YOUR HEALTH

Getting your first UTI can be really scary. If you feel shame about it, or about its ties to sexual activity, that can keep you from getting the help you need. Remember that UTIs have many causes, and that there's no shame in taking responsibility for your health.

There are many challenges in the treatment of urinary tract infections for both health-care professionals and patients. Doctors have to make decisions about prescribing antibiotics. Patients need to learn about their infections so they can treat themselves effectively and prevent themselves from getting another infection.

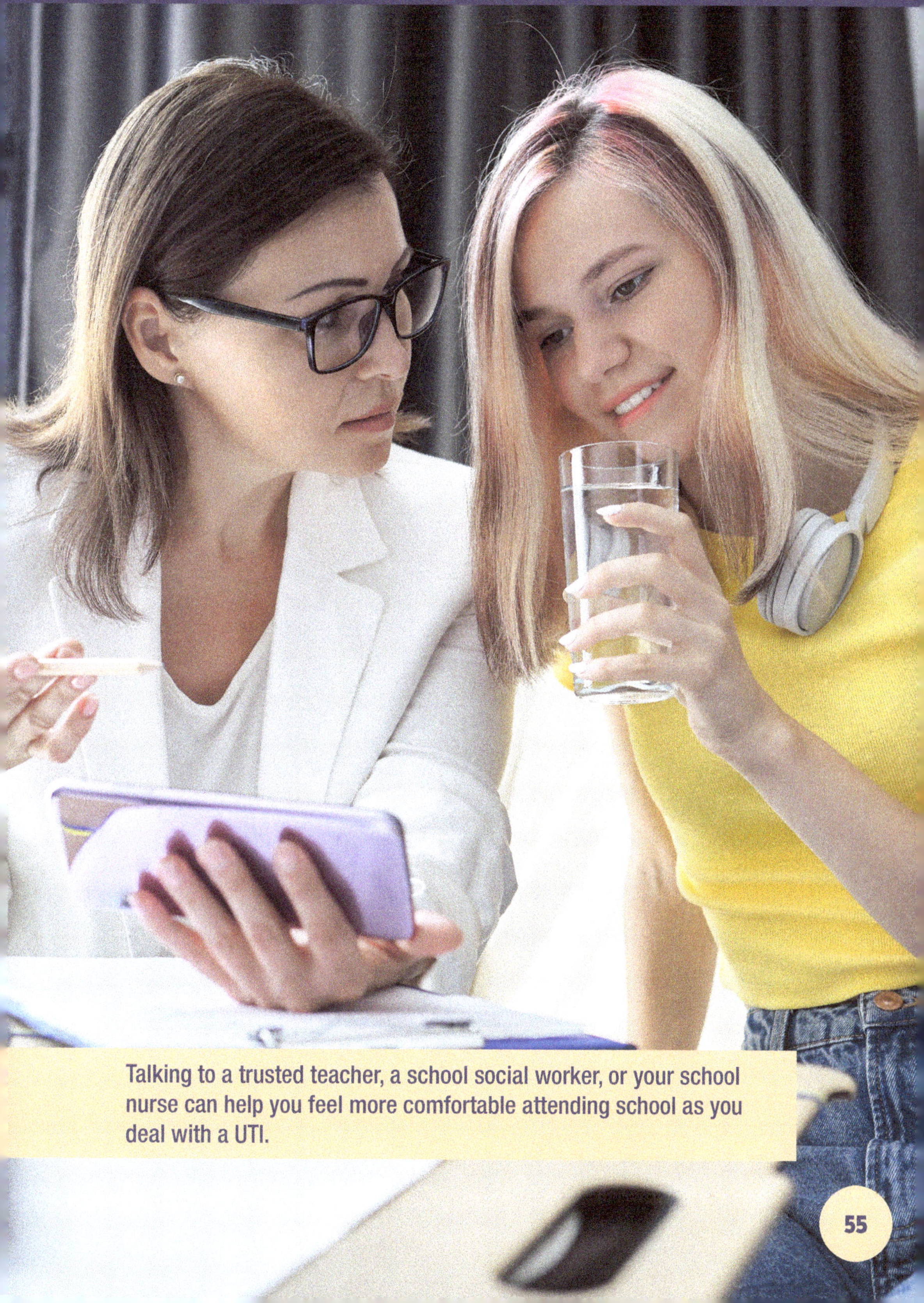

Talking to a trusted teacher, a school social worker, or your school nurse can help you feel more comfortable attending school as you deal with a UTI.

GLOSSARY

abnormality Something that is not normal.

advocate To support or argue for something.

circulation Orderly movement within a system.

contagious Able to spread infection or disease from one being to another.

contraception Something that prevents pregnancy; birth control.

diagnose To recognize a disease by signs and symptoms.

diaphragm A domed rubber device placed over the cervix to prevent conception.

diverticula Sacs that branch off from canals or cavities.

hygiene Conditions or practices that are good for one's health.

microbe An organism too small to be seen by the unaided eye.

obstruct To block or close up by an obstacle.

prescription A written direction, often by a doctor, for use of treatments such as medicine.

prevalence The degree to which something happens often; the percentage of a population that is affected with a particular disease at a given time.

probiotic A microorganism that when consumed maintains or restores beneficial bacteria to the digestive tract.

puberty The state or period of first becoming capable of reproducing sexually.

severity The degree of being bad, serious, unpleasant, or harsh.

spasm An involuntary and abnormal muscular contraction.

specimen A portion or quantity of material for testing, examining, or studying something.

stagnant Without inflow or outflow; stale.

sterile Free from living organisms, especially harmful bacteria or viruses.

stigma A mark of shame or discredit.

symptom Something that indicates the existence of a certain disease or condition.

supplement Something consumed in addition to a person's diet.

susceptible Open or unresistant to something, such as a disease.

toxin Any poison produced by an organism, such as bacteria.

transgender Referring to a person whose gender identity is different from that usually associated with the anatomy they were born with.

vaccine A shot that keeps a person from getting a certain sickness.

virus A microscopic agent that causes infection in cells.

water-soluble Able to dissolve in water.

FOR MORE INFORMATION

The Center for Young Women's Health
Boston Children's Hospital League's Resource Center
333 Longwood Ave, 5th Floor
Boston, MA 02115
Twitter: @CYWH
YouTube: CYWHBoston
The Center for Young Women's Health provides teens and young adults with sexual health information and education programs. It's a collaboration between the Division of Adolescent and Young Adult Medicine and the Division of Gynecology at Boston Children's Hospital.

Healthy Teen Network
1501 Saint Paul Street, Suite 114
Baltimore, MD 21202
Website: www.healthyteennetwork.org
Instagram: @healthyteennetwork
Twitter: @healthyteen
This organization works to advance social change, connect teens, and empower teens to protect their health and be more aware of sexual health issues.

National Coalition for Sexual Health
Website: nationalcoalitionforsexualhealth.org
Instagram: @nationalcoalitionsexualhealth
Twitter: @NCSH_
This coalition works together to improve sexual health of Americans, make sexual health a part of normal conversation, and spread accurate sexual health information.

National Women's Health Network
1413 K Street NW, 4th Floor
Washington, D.C. 20005
(202) 682-2640
Website: nwhn.org
Instagram: @thenwhn
Twitter: @TheNWHN
The National Women's Health Network is a national initiative that works for health advocacy and provides high-quality information about female health concerns.

Planned Parenthood
Phone: 1-800-230-PLAN
Website: www.plannedparenthood.org
Instagram: @plannedparenthood
Twitter: @PPFA
Planned Parenthood is a nonprofit organization that provides sexual and reproductive health care, sexual education, and accurate information on sexual health to people around the world.

Women's Health Matters
76 Grenville St, 4th Floor
Toronto, ON, Canada
Website: www.womenshealthmatters.ca
Twitter: @WHealthMatters
This Canadian foundation provides a trusted source of information, news, and research on many women's health issues, through the Women's College Hospital.

FOR FURTHER READING

Benson, Alana. *Everything You Need to Know About Birth Control.* New York, NY: Rosen Publishing, 2019.

DeCarlo, Carolyn. *Everything You Need to Know About the Risks of Unprotected Sex.* New York, NY: Rosen Publishing, 2019.

De Witte, Christina. *The Ultimate Survival Guide to Being a Girl: On Love, Body Image, School, and Making It Through Life.* Philadelphia, PA: Running Press Kids, 2018.

Gonzales, Katheryn, and Karen Rayne PhD. *Trans+: Love, Sex, Romance, and Being You.* Washington, DC: Magination Press, 2019.

Hope, Michelle, and Amy Lang. *The Girls' Guide to Sex Education: Over 100 Honest Answers to Urgent Questions about Puberty, Relationships, and Growing Up.* Emeryville, CA: Rockridge Press, 2018.

Lang, Jennifer. *Consent: The New Rules of Sex Education: Every Teen's Guide to Healthy Sexual Relationships.* San Antonio, TX: Althea Press, 2018.

Langford, Jo. *The Pride Guide: A Guide to Sexual and Social Health for LGBTQ Youth.* Lanham, MD: Rowman & Littlefield, 2018.

Leff, Carrie, Dr., and Dr. Lisa Klein. *Celebrate Your Body 2: The Ultimate Puberty Book for Preteen and Teen Girls.* Emeryville, CA: Rockridge Press, 2019.

Moem, Erika, and Matthew Nolan. *Let's Talk About It: The Teen's Guide to Sex, Relationships, and Being a Human.* New York, NY: Random House Graphic, 2021.

Wolny, Philip. *I Have an STD. Now What?* New York, NY: Rosen Publishing, 2015.

INDEX

A

B

C

D

E

F

G

PHOTO CREDITS

Cover and chapter heads Kateryna Kon/Shutterstock.com; series background Lu Vesper; p. 4 Ann Patchanan/Shutterstock.com; pp. 6, 21, 41 Monkey Business Images/Shutterstock.com; p. 8 Albina Gavrilovic/Shutterstock.com; p. 9 Designua/Shutterstock.com; p. 10 Total art/Shutterstock.com; p. 13 Andrey_Popov/Shutterstock.com; p. 15 AnnaStills/Shutterstock.com; p. 20 Diego Cervo/Shutterstock.com; pp. 23, 46 fizkes/Shutterstock.com; p. 25 lithian/Shutterstock.com; p. 28 siamionau pavel/Shutterstock.com; p. 30 S_Photo/Shutterstock.com; p. 32 Pablo Rasero/Shutterstock.com; p. 34 Lightfield Studios/Shutterstock.com; p. 35 SofikoS/Shutterstock.com; p. 38 Iakov Filimonov/Shutterstock.com; p. 40 B-D-S Piotr Marcinski/Shutterstock.com; p. 47 Darren Baker/Shutterstock.com; p. 48 Eo naya/Shutterstock.com; p. 51 AppleZoomZoom/Shutterstock.com; p. 55 VH-studio/Shutterstock.com.

Designer: Michael Flynn
Editor: Caitie McAneney